Take the Fight Out of Food

HOW TO PREVENT AND SOLVE YOUR CHILD'S EATING PROBLEMS

Donna Fish, M.S., L.C.S.W.

**FOR CHILDREN AGED NINE
MONTHS THROUGH NINE YEARS**

ATRIA BOOKS

NEW YORK • LONDON • TORONTO • SYDNEY

ATRIA BOOKS
1230 Avenue of the Americas
New York, NY 10020

Library of Congress Cataloging-in-Publication Data

Fish, Donna.
　　Take the fight out of food : how to prevent and solve your
child's eating problems : for children aged nine months
through nine years / Donna Fish.—1st Atria Books trade
pbk. ed.
　　　　p.　cm.
　　Includes bibliographical references and index.
　　ISBN 978-0-7434-7779-6
　　1. Eating disorders in children.　2. Children—Nutrition—
Psychological aspects.　3. Diet therapy for children.　I. Title.

RJ506.E18F55　2005
618.92'8526—dc22

2004062903

First Atria Books trade paperback edition May 2005

1　3　5　7　9　10　8　6　4　2

ATRIA BOOKS is a trademark of Simon & Schuster, Inc.

Manufactured in the United States of America

For information regarding special discounts for bulk purchases,
please contact Simon & Schuster Special Sales at 1-800-456-6798
or business@simonandschuster.com

To my girls, Nicole Alexandra, Sophie Antonia, and Lulu Hattie Davis, and to all of our children: may you always eat with gusto, passion, and enjoyment. Here's to freedom with food!

Contents

Foreword   *ix*

Introduction   *xiii*

PART ONE—EATING FOR LIFE
STARTS WITH PARENTS

Chapter One Separating Our Own Food
Attitudes from Our Children's Eating Behaviors

3

Chapter Two Factor In Your Child's
Developmental Stage

36

Chapter Three Identify Your Child's Eating Style

57

PART TWO—THE FOUR STEPS OF
EATING FOR LIFE

Chapter Four Step One: Talk to Your Kids
About Nutrition

85

Contents

Chapter Five Step Two: Reboot the Connection
Between the Belly and the Head
119

Chapter Six Step Three: Separate Hunger and Fullness
from Other Feelings
141

Chapter Seven Step Four: Teach Your Child to Become
a Confident Decision Maker
160

PART THREE—ESTABLISHING PARAMETERS
THAT WORK FOR YOU

Chapter Eight Finding Your Comfort Zone
191

Chapter Nine Commonly Asked Questions
and Answers
214

Resources 235
Bibliography 237
Acknowledgments 241
Index 247

Foreword

Ask any pediatrician what parents are most concerned with during well-child visits and he or she will say that while no objective studies exist, the most common questions asked by parents are about feeding. When children are born, parents' questions include "Should I breast- or bottle-feed?" and "Am I giving too much milk or too little?" Then, during the toddler years, the questions change to "Why does my child just play with his food?" and "Why doesn't he like to eat green vegetables?" These questions about how to best feed their children persist—regardless of the age or gender of the child, age of the parents, or socioeconomic level of the family. Every grandmother wants a chubby-cheeked grandchild. Every mother wants her child to eat all his vegetables.

Yet, all this said, it is clear that children's diets must be managed. Toddlers and children are exposed to a variety of foods: some healthy, some with very little nutritional value. Parents can provide their children with only "healthy" foods, but ultimately the parents can't make their kids eat. It's a difficult battle.

Foreword

In this book, Donna Fish provides the twenty-first-century family with a sensible, practical approach to this common family problem. She shows us how to artfully balance the pressures of eating right, limiting sweets, not creating eating disorders, and still enjoying the time with our children.

Donna's life experiences give her a unique perspective on this issue. Previously a dancer, she knows firsthand the overwhelming pressures of being and staying thin and fit. Now a psychotherapist, her vocation demands realistic answers to problems. And, of course, having three daughters, trying to balance the pressures of being a "good" yet working mother is paramount in her thoughts. As you read this book you can feel the calming, reassuring style that has evolved from her background.

Take the Fight Out of Food begins with parents exploring their own feelings and thoughts toward food and feeding practices, many of which stem from the parents' upbringing. (Interestingly, I find that grandparents put subtle pressure on their offspring as to child-rearing practices. In my office, most grandmothers report that *their* children had never whined about food, always sat quietly during mealtimes, and, of course, ate all of the food on their plate — without making a mess and regardless of the child's age.) The book goes on to review the different developmental ages of children and their particular eating styles. With each example, parents are given a sensible approach and practical steps to deal with the food issues of their child. Then comes the description and discussion of the six main types of eaters. My favorite is "The Beige Food Eater." In my almost thirty years as a pediatrician, the beige food eater demonstrates the most common eating pattern throughout childhood. This aversion to any food with color begins at about fifteen to eighteen months of age and runs through late childhood. The child at nine months of age is an angel. Breakfast is cereal and fruit. Lunch is full-fat yogurt with a sippy cup of water. Dinner includes chicken with a generous amount of green and yellow vegetables. At this age, kids even like spicy foods! But then everything changes. This sweet infant grows up and turns into the *terrible two!* Suddenly, only foods of certain bland color and consistency will be consumed. Milk, cheese, bread, Cheerios, and chicken nuggets are fine, but fruits and vegetables are not. Even when those "colored" foods are embedded in omelets or pasta, the green foods are simply picked out and discarded from the plate or serving tray. What could be more frustrating for the parents who only want their child to grow up big and strong and to enjoy the pleasures of vegetables?

Donna handles the parents with skill, a calming voice, and practical advice. Remember, that in this culture, 99 percent of children will still get adequate nutrition. Continue to model by example, and serve and eat vegetables. Enjoy mealtime, don't dread it. If you're still concerned, ask your pediatrician about adding multivitamins with iron to your child's diet.

Take the Fight Out of Food: How to Prevent and Solve Your Child's Eating Problems is a *must read* for every busy family struggling with mealtimes.

Michael Traister, M.D.
Clinical Associate Professor of Pediatrics
New York University School of Medicine

Private Practice, New York City

Introduction

I AM A MOTHER of three daughters. I am also a psychotherapist with a fifteen-year practice working with adults and children on various emotional and psychological issues. I am also a former dancer. But it is by and large the mother in me that has fueled my passion to write this book about how to help our children develop a healthy relationship with food. My goal is to share a program that has already been successful for hundreds of my patients so that many more children and their parents can learn to navigate the often confusing information about diet and food with which we are bombarded every day of the year. Essentially, I want to help parents teach kids how to eat in a rational, enjoyable way by providing them with the building blocks of what I call "eating for life."

As a woman, I am aware of the pressures all of us feel to look good, be thin and fit, and eat healthy foods. In my "previous life" as a professional dancer, I struggled with yo-yo dieting for many years. Was I overweight? No, but I always thought I needed to lose another five to ten pounds for an audition, a performance, or simply so that I would feel better about my body. How I ate overshadowed my life, determining daily how I felt about myself. If I had successfully stayed away from foods that were fattening or "bad" for me, it was a "good" day. If I ate too much chocolate, bread, or pasta, it was a "bad" day.

When I changed careers and got to wear "real" clothing (which can hide a multitude of sins!), I instantly felt less pressure to lose that stubborn five or ten pounds, but I was still obsessed with food and eating. Finally, however, I began to experiment with eating a range of foods, including those I had always thought of as fattening or bad. I started to allow myself that chocolate bar after my sandwich at lunch, the toast with butter in the morning, and a second slice of pizza when I was really hungry. My new rule was to eat whatever I wanted until I felt full and sated. I made a conscious decision not to use food as either a reward or a punishment. And the more I allowed myself to eat whatever I wanted, the more in tune with my body I became. Soon I was able to ask myself such questions as, "Do I really want all of this chocolate bar or just a few bites?" Knowing I could eat more later if I wished, I often decided that a bite or two was enough. Sometimes I ate the whole thing, but the more I allowed myself the freedom to choose what I truly wanted, the less I was preoccupied with food. In time, I was eating all foods in moderation, and ironically, I lost those ten pounds I had always fretted about.

You may be saying to yourself, "Oh, but I could never do that—I'm addicted to chocolate" (or to bread, or to pasta). Perhaps, but by teaching many people how to think about food differently and, as a result, eat differently, I have helped them get over attachments to favorite foods, even when they believed they had no control. After acquiring a new set of rules for eating, men, women, and children can completely change their eating habits and relationship to food.

But what does all of this have to do with teaching children how to become good eaters? Although I have now worked in the field of eating disorders for more than fifteen years, it was about ten years ago that I began to help parents resolve their concerns about their children and food: "My child isn't eating enough"; "My child is eating too much"; "My child takes after her father, who is overweight. I worry she will have a weight problem, too, but I don't know how to handle it without making her feel bad"; "My partner and I fight all the time; he thinks I'm letting the kids have too much sugar, but I don't think it's such a big deal"; "My child won't eat one single vegetable; how on earth will she get the proper nutrition?!"

As a parent reading this book, you too may have had these or other concerns, because as parents we know that ultimately our children, regardless of their eating style or behavior, will need to be able to make decisions about food on their own. All of us want our children to have a healthy relationship with food, and we certainly want them to be able to take good care of their bodies when they are no longer under our wing. In short, we want them to eat for life. We want them to be able to figure out whether they should have an extra helping of dessert or fill up on more protein. We would like them to eat in moderation—to eat when they are hungry and to stop when they are full. We want them to know how to negotiate sugar and junk food. Sure, there is a movement to provide healthier lunches and get rid of vending machines in schools, but we still want to be confident that our son knows how to eat a range of foods to keep himself strong and healthy. Or that our daughter, who is entering puberty, an age when many girls are at higher risk for developing an eating disorder, has confidence in her ability to eat the foods she loves in moderation. These are the tools your children will be integrating into their lives as they learn to eat for life.

As you help your children know their bodies and know themselves, they will learn—with your guidance and through trial and error—which foods work for them and which do not. I always say to my children, "You are the expert on your own body, and it is your job to pay close attention to it and take care of it. Nobody but you knows when you are hungry or full, and what that feels like. Nobody but you knows what your body may feel like eating, so it is up to you to know how to feed it well." I teach my clients, both adults and children, that all food is good, but different foods do different things to you and for you. The key, therefore, is to maintain balance, which means eating a range of foods, so that your body receives all the essential nutrients (protein, carbohydrates, and, yes, even fat!) it needs to grow and be strong and help you concentrate. And equally important are the desserts or treats that make your tongue and spirit happy. When children learn how to eat within this basic framework, they can handle days here and there of emotional eating or overeating—and so can we! Indeed, it's crucial that parents allow such flexibility—for both our children and ourselves.

Take the Fight Out of Food will not only provide you with the tools you need to instill these building blocks of good eating in your children, but it will also help you maintain that all-important balance between being involved in how and what your children are eating and becoming so overinvolved that you are always making decisions for them or trying to fix their behavior. You will learn how to establish realistic standards that make you comfortable and that your children are able to follow.

By looking at your own food history, you will begin to see the connection between your own attitudes toward food and your children's eating behavior. I have found time and again that if parents have set unrealistic standards for themselves, they can unwittingly communicate that misinformation to their children. Children are keen observers and instinctually pick up on our own feelings about food. So even if we try hard never to say "Do I look fat?" in front of our daughters, they do know how we eat and how we think about ourselves. This book will help you recognize your own food issues and concerns, and help you to figure out whether or not your attitudes are affecting your children's eating behavior. The answers may surprise you.

Take the Fight Out of Food offers a program that works. The four steps I provide for teaching kids how to eat for life have already helped hundreds of parents relax more and worry less, and they can do the same for you. You will learn how to resolve problematic eating behaviors with solutions that are practical and easy to implement. And as you navigate through these problems, you will be putting into place the tools your children need to prevent future problems, which is the essence of teaching them how to eat for life. By doing that, you will feel increased confidence in yourself as a parent, as well as increase your children's confidence in themselves as they gradually learn to take responsibility for feeding their bodies. As the fight is taken out of food, dinnertime will become a fun, bonding time when your family can sit down and be together.

Teaching your kids how to eat for life is actually quite simple. First you gather information—about yourself, your children's developmental stage, and eating style. Then you turn to your kids and apply the four steps of eating for life:

Step One: Talk to your kids about nutrition.

Step Two: Reboot the connection between the belly and the head.

Step Three: Separate hunger and fullness from other feelings.

Step Four: Teach your child to become a confident decision maker.

To help you complete these steps, I'll provide not only hands-on exercises you can use immediately but also tips on how to continue fostering an "eat for life" attitude in your kids throughout their childhood and into their adulthood. And then, finally, you will determine how to establish the rules and parameters that best suit your family and your individual children.

Remember, you are the expert on your own children. You know their likes, their dislikes, their temperament, and their stage of development. When you apply this information to the four steps I'll be teaching, you will be able to give them all the tools they need to establish a healthy relationship with food—for life.

PART ONE

Eating for Life Starts with Parents

CHAPTER ONE

Separating Our Own Food Attitudes from Our Children's Eating Behaviors

As soon as my daughter could walk, my mother started to comment on her chunky legs. "You better watch her, Carly, you don't want her to get fat." For goodness sake, my daughter is only two!

CARLY, MOTHER OF TWO

My mother raised me to eat when I was hungry and stop eating when I was full. I am convinced that what she taught me has saved my life. As a professional actress I have watched both men and women in my field literally starve to death to maintain the body they think the entertainment world is looking for.

SAMANTHA, ACTRESS AND MOTHER OF ONE

HUNDREDS OF PARENTS, who are struggling with or worried about how their children are eating, have told me poignant stories about how critical they are of their own eating habits. And often, once I prompt them to examine the attitudes with which they were raised, they report that they have always felt they were either failing themselves by eating too much or making bad choices, or failing their parents because they didn't eat enough of the "food of love" they were offered.

If there's one thing I've learned from listening to these stories, it's that there is a direct connection between parents' food attitudes and how they deal with their kids' eating behaviors. As one mother told me, "I have an easier time talking about sex with my kids than food. My mother was so controlling and involved with my food that I always felt I was failing and ended up with a real weight problem. I still struggle with weight and my relationship to food, and because of that, I am terrified to interfere with how my kids eat. I feel paralyzed when it comes to saying anything at all about nutrition." Acknowledging and understanding this connection between our own food attitudes and our children's eating behaviors is the first step toward teaching our kids how to eat for life. And yet it's also one of the most challenging steps because it requires that we look at our own food history and eating experiences.

In this chapter, you will revisit your family food legacy and the tape loops (or food attitudes) this early experience created. As you become more familiar with your own food attitudes, you will automatically become better able to separate your own experience from what is going on with your children. Indeed, you may discover that what you perceive as your children's eating problems are really not problems at all, but rather styles of eating that are simply different from your own.

Taking the Fight Out of Food:
Whose Problem Is It?

One of the most common complaints I hear from parents is that mealtime is one long power struggle. "My two-and-a-half-year-old won't sit in his high chair!" "My four-year-old incessantly demands dessert!" "My three-year-old throws a fit if I don't give her a cookie!" Parents come into my office completely at their wits' end.

In one such case, a mother came to see me because she could not understand her three-year-old son's picky eating behavior. Jennifer is thirty-six, with an engaging wit and the ability to turn even the most mundane incident into a stand-up comedy routine. She always has a twinkle in her eye and has a lot of great ideas about feeding children. Indeed, she knows that when she "lets go and relaxes" around food, her kids relax and eat better. Her first son (she has two) was a "foodie" like her. He loved exploring new foods and ate almost anything she offered, which is why Jennifer was surprised by her younger son's food issues. From day one, he was a very picky eater and often simply refused to eat at all. When she consulted her pediatrician, however, he assured her that her son was perfectly healthy and right where he should be in terms of growth. His advice was simply to "back off" and "let him be."

But even though knowing her son was in good health helped to allay Jennifer's fear that he would end up with scurvy, she still could not ignore everything she'd heard about encouraging him to eat. It was very difficult for her to sit by and watch her son refuse food.

Jennifer's reaction is not very different from that of

many parents whose feelings of competence come from nurturing and feeding their children. When our children eat, we have concrete evidence that we are doing a good job, helping them make their way in the world with strong, healthy bodies. And when they don't eat well, or we *think* they are not eating well, we assume we must be doing a bad job. But we still need to ask, What was really going on between Jennifer and her son? What was the problem? Was it hers or her son's?

The first thing Jennifer and I did was to look at her own food legacy, and when we did that, we soon discovered that Jennifer had been raised as a dieter from the time she was very young. (Her joke is that her formative experience with religion was Weight Watchers, since she was sent by her mother at the age of nine to meetings that were held at the temple!) After years of diet camps and therapy to help resolve her food issues, she had come to terms with a way of eating that felt comfortable, and she was thrilled to be a mother who could let her sons enjoy their food. She was not going to repeat her own mother's mistakes by restricting what they ate.

So when Todd began refusing to eat, Jennifer found herself trying to fight back, almost force-feeding him, and frequently becoming angry at his resistance to her carefully prepared meals. She wanted him to eat and enjoy his food, but she was unwittingly contributing to the fight: the more she encouraged Todd to eat, the more he resisted.

Despite thinking that she handled food differently from her restricting mother, Jennifer gradually began to realize that, in her own way, and despite having the opposite goal, she was being just as controlling as her mother had been. At first, all she could see was her son's resistance to her efforts to help him. When he would "simply not listen," Jennifer reacted—sometimes in anger, sometimes out of anxiety and frustration. It took a while for her to see that her reaction was actually fueling the power struggle with her son.

Once she realized that, we were able to address her need to give up trying to control the situation, so that she would be better able to let go of the outcome. Meanwhile, at a deeper level, she also began to separate her own fear of being restricted (a holdover from her mother's attempts to restrict her own food intake) from her son's seemingly self-restricting behavior. Only then could she see that Todd was, in fact, reacting to the pressure she was putting on him to eat. When Jennifer backed off, Todd began to eat more regularly—though never with the same adventurousness as his older brother.

Children—at any age—seem to be masters at detecting our agendas: they know exactly what we want them to do and then often do just the opposite. What is our agenda when it comes to food? We simply want our children to eat well—that is, eat the food we have lovingly and painstakingly put before them. And know this: even if you think you're being discreet, cheerful, or absolutely blasé as you serve breakfast, lunch, or dinner, even a ten-month-old in his high chair can detect your concern, worry, and anxiety that he get that broccoli down the hatch.

I met Carolyn when she attended one of my workshops because she was concerned about her nine-year-old son, who had become quite overweight. She herself had struggled with a weight problem in the past and resolved it by sticking to a diet that was totally free of sugar and junk food. She herself ate plenty of fresh fruits and vegetables, and every meal she prepared for her two sons was made up of a variety of nutritious, organic foods.

Although her younger son seemed to enjoy whatever she put in front of him, the older child wanted only starchy carbohydrates, such as potatoes, pasta, and bread. He wouldn't touch vegetables and also fought with her to eat chocolate bars and other sweets, none of which Carolyn allowed in the house. From the time he was two, she told me, their every interaction about food had been adversarial. Now she was even more worried because he was really gaining weight and clearly hoarding the foods she'd never allowed him to have.

As we explored the situation, two issues became clear: one was that Carolyn had a food legacy associated with very health-conscious eating that went back three generations. Her mother and grandmother had both eaten only "healthful" foods and had restricted foods deemed "bad." The other was that both Carolyn and her mother had weight problems and frequently felt guilty about how much they ate. Her mother was not happy with her figure and had constantly berated herself for failing to restrict her food intake. She also criticized Carolyn when she was growing up by focusing on her weight. In fact, Carolyn said that when she returned from a trip to India, during which she had become very ill with dysentery, her mother had joked that she looked great because she had lost so much weight.

Like her mother, Carolyn believed that in order to be a good parent she had to make sure her children ate nutritiously ALL THE TIME. And because of this food legacy,

Carolyn felt completely stymied by her older son's eating behavior and had no tools for dealing with his determination to make his own decisions about food.

Did he, in fact, have an eating problem? Or was he simply reacting to Carolyn's rigidity about food and eating? Had her son internalized his mother's fears about gaining weight? These were the questions Carolyn and I began to unravel as we worked together. Indeed, once Carolyn saw how her food legacy had affected her own eating habits and attitudes toward food, she began to realize that her son's weight gain had triggered her fear—not that he would become fat but that she herself could not control her own food intake. Once she was able to be more objective about her fears and associations with food and weight, she was better able to deal with her son's situation. In the end, Carolyn decided to try to be more flexible, allowing her son to have some sweets and candy. Predictably, once she made these foods available instead of forbidden, her son stopped hoarding them. And as Carolyn began teaching him how certain foods impacted his body, he began—slowly but surely—to try vegetables and protein to round out his diet. As you will see in the upcoming chapters, even the most willful children can learn how to increase their range of foods—if they are taught in a palatable manner.

What Is Your Family Food Legacy?

Most negative attitudes toward food begin at home. Therefore as you prepare to help your children become good eaters, you need to be clear about the kind of environment in which you were raised. Use the questions below as a way to consider the rules, tone, and values that pertained to eating in your family.

1. Did your parents ever tell you to stop eating before you felt you were full?
2. Did either of your parents ever pressure you to go on a diet?
3. Did a friend ever show you how to diet?
4. Was anyone in your household ever on a diet when you were growing up?
5. Did anyone binge and/or restrict foods in a regular way?
6. Did anyone "eat like a bird," always picking at food and never sitting down and enjoying a meal?
7. Did your mother, father, or any of your siblings go from diet to diet, always trying to lose weight but never feeling comfortable with their body image?
8. Were their diets successful only temporarily?
9. Did you eat predominantly "healthy" food?
10. Did your family eat a lot of bread, pasta, and other starchy foods?
11. Did your family consume a lot of fried food?
12. Did your parents let you snack on junk food?
13. Did your family keep soda in the house?
14. Were there any foods that were forbidden or only served on very special occasions?
15. Was there an emphasis in your household on making sure you ate enough?
16. Do you come from a culture in which food was scarce and, as a result, eating was believed to assure health and happiness?

There are no right or wrong answers to these questions. Rather they are intended to help you become more aware of how you were raised with relation to food. They are not intended to evoke either blame or self-praise. As a general rule, your food legacy will fall into one of four categories.

1. You were raised in an environment where food was equated with love. Such an environment can create a situation in which you might feel that you are letting someone down if you don't eat all the food she or he has prepared. It can also lead you to use food to process emotions rather than to deal with your feelings directly.

2. You were raised in a restrictive environment where the types and amounts of food you ate were closely monitored by your parents. Often this environment is characterized by dieting and maintaining weight and tends to evoke one of two reactions: either you were comfortable with these restrictions and want the same for your kids, or, once out of your parents' control you rebelled, eating whatever you wanted without regard to nutrition or balance, which could make you uncomfortable with setting limits and establishing parameters around food and eating for your children.

3. You were raised in an environment where one or more of your family members went on restrictive diets and lost weight only later to regain it. Such a legacy may cause you to believe that you are not in control of food, which can then lead to restrictive/binge behavior and yo-yo dieting.

4. You were raised in an environment where meals were enjoyed, a variety of foods was offered, and there was

little or no emphasis on how much or how little one should eat of any particular food. Meals usually consisted of a balance among healthy nutritious foods, with an allowance for some sugar or junk food. There was an emphasis on eating for enjoyment instead of a focus on rigidity. This environment is the most likely to produce a healthy attitude toward food and eating.

Whichever environment you were raised in, it is likely that you have internalized your legacy, and that it has subtly but powerfully influenced your present attitudes toward food. It is these internalized, unconscious food attitudes, or what I call tape loops, that can unwittingly influence the way you are dealing with your own kids about food.

What Are Your Tape Loops?

Examining and disrupting your tape loops, those voices in your head fueled by your attitudes toward food and eating, is the next step toward separating your own food attitudes from your children's behaviors. Have you ever heard a voice in your head berating you when you ate that second piece of cake, and then said to yourself, "Now I have really blown it! I am totally off my usual diet, and I better not eat anything tomorrow." The internalized attitude that you don't have control over what or how much you eat helps create the feeling that you have "blown it," leaving you at risk for deciding that the only way to compensate is to not eat anything at all the next day. When you begin to restrict what you eat, you put yourself at risk for creating or continuing a restrict-binge-restrict cycle. What happens with such an attitude? You may eat two, then maybe three pieces of cake, and the chips, and then the cookies, and the ice cream, and whatever other food you deem "bad."

Indeed, experts are now beginning to understand that this negative cycle impacts metabolism and can result in

Just the Thought of Restricting Induces Overeating

SEVERAL STUDIES HAVE BEEN DONE on the effects of rigid dieting on actual eating behavior and consequent weight gain. Herman and Mack (1975) studied women who were very concerned with eating, dieting, and weight and observed that anytime they thought they had blown their diets and broken from their rigid dietary standards, they resorted to "all or none" thinking, which in turn provoked binge eating. Furthermore, the women in the study demonstrated an inability to feel full. If they thought that they had gone off their diet, they not only were unable to detect their signal of fullness but also consumed—at minimum—twice as much food as women who were not on rigid diets.

And, Spencer and Fremouw (1979) observed that women who merely *thought* they had blown their diets took in more calories than others. The study concluded that chronic avoidance of food resulted in overeating, weight gain, and increased body fat. It is now widely understood in the field of eating problems that "the best defense against binge eating is to eat" (Johnson and Connors, 1987). I always say in my practice, "A chocolate bar a day keeps the fat away!"

The Domino Effect of Yo-Yo Dieting and Restricting Food

IN 1950, ANSEL KEYS and his colleagues studied the effects of starvation by severely limiting the food intake of a group of normal healthy men. Prior to the study, these men had no emotional problems or any issues with food. However, during the period of restriction, the men demonstrated profound social, emotional, cognitive, and physiological changes. They became depressed and withdrawn. They were extraordinarily preoccupied with thoughts of food. And their metabolisms slowed down. During the refeeding phase, most of the men gained weight and significantly increased their percentage of body fat. Many could not lose this weight, and even eight months after the refeeding phase, one-third of them remained seriously preoccupied with food, had eating problems, and retained an increased percentage of body fat.

weight gain rather than weight loss. During a binge, the body responds to the influx of food by storing body fat, as if readying itself for a future famine.

This physiologic reaction is the reason why people with a history of yo-yo dieting can end up regaining more weight than they lost. With each attempt to lose weight, they begin to trigger the mechanism that leads to storing more and more fat. Scientific research supports the idea that people who chronically restrict their food intake not only disrupt their metabolism and wind up gaining more weight and a percentage of body fat but also become more preoccupied with thoughts about food. For more on the metabolic impact of yo-yo dieting see Debra Waterhouse's book *Outsmarting the Female Fat Cell.*

Another tape loop might lead to your needing to feed your children in order to make you feel that you are loving them enough. People who come from backgrounds that emphasized eating as a way to show community within the family as well as love and appreciation for the chef (frequently the mother) often carry tape loops that cause anxiety if a child doesn't eat "enough." They might fear that

Endocrine Changes as a Result of Dieting in Young Women

IN 1984, FICHTER AND PIRKE did a study in which a group of young women were asked to restrict their food intake for six weeks. The results showed profound endocrine disturbances that did not resolve themselves until the women returned to their normal weight. The physiological changes included an elevation of the plasma cortisol levels (which negatively impact the body's ability to manage stress), an increase in growth hormone levels, and a decrease in hormone-stimulating levels. What these results tell us is that even one incidence of severe dieting or restriction can have profound physiological effects on a young person's body. Keep this information in mind the next time you overhear a nine-year-old girl wanting to go on her first diet. Some children may indeed need to lose weight, but they must be guided by a healthy, rational plan.

their children won't be healthy, that their children don't love them, or that they themselves are not being good parents.

These tape loops, as I've said, are a direct result of the internalized messages created by your family food legacy. Consider these four general attitudes toward food:

1. You tend to eat when you are feeling stressed, anxious, bored, lonely, or in need of comfort. You use food to celebrate an event or to reward yourself.
2. You categorize foods as either good or bad, which often causes you to be preoccupied with closely monitoring what you are eating on a daily basis.
3. You feel you don't have control over food or eating; you are prone to dieting and/or restrictive/binge behavior.
4. You don't think about food. You eat when you are hungry, reaching for whatever is around and available. You are not overly concerned with nutrition or eating in moderation because you trust that your body is getting the nutrients it needs for optimal health and well-being.

If your general attitude toward food is characterized by either (1), (2), or (3), you have internalized a negative attitude toward eating, which may in turn be determining how you are dealing with your children's eating behavior. On the other hand, if you feel your attitude is most akin to that described in (4), you more than likely have a healthy, objective way of addressing your children's eating issues. In essence, tape loops—whether they voice admonishments to eat more or eat less—can interfere with your ability to deal with your children's eating behaviors objectively and clearly. Therefore, you need to become aware of your own tape loops and separate them from your children's behavior with food.

How Your Tape Loops May Be Affecting Your Children

Not surprisingly, there is a direct correlation between how parents treat themselves and how they treat their children: parents who are more relaxed about how they eat will be more relaxed about how their children eat. These parents will also have an easier time if the pediatrician tells them to "back off" when they begin to worry about their toddler who never seems to eat anything, or about their five-year-old who eats only peanut butter and jelly sandwiches.

Parents usually fall somewhere on a spectrum of attitudes about eating. At one extreme is a very rigid approach toward what foods their kids should eat, and at the other extreme is allowing kids to eat anything that interests them. If you have a hard time forgiving yourself after eating fattening foods, then you might have a hard time relaxing when your children eat those foods, and you might worry if they have days when they eat mostly cake and ice cream. On the other hand, if you are relaxed about food and have never dieted a day in your life, you might not even give a second thought to your child's sugar intake. You might focus on other things, like getting him to sleep so he will wake up feeling fresh in the morning. The more easygoing you are about the way you eat, the easier it will be for you to go with the ebb and flow of your child's eating because you will be confident that his nutritional needs are being met. Indeed, as you will see in chapter four, pediatricians and nutritionists agree that for children nutrition is achieved on a two-week basis, not day to day.

Let's see how flexible or rigid you are about eating, and how that corresponds to your response to your child's eating behavior.

1. Visualize a line that contains four points, A, B, C, and D.

A	B	C	D

2. Imagine that you are attending your best friend's fortieth birthday party, where your favorite birthday cake is served. You:

   A. Look at it and say to yourself, "I am definitely not having a piece; I cannot do that!"

   B. Take one piece after deliberating for ten minutes, and it tastes so good that you have another half. You then figure you blew it, so you might as well have three more pieces, and then you move on to eating the other foods you didn't taste because you *know* you will not have this stuff again starting tomorrow.

   C. You eat the piece of cake but spend a lot of the evening feeling fat and thinking about how you shouldn't have done that and you certainly won't have any more fattening food.

   D. You have and enjoy the cake, knowing that one piece of cake will not affect your weight.

3. Imagine that your beautiful baby is now ten months old, you are still nursing a bit, and you find that you are also still struggling to lose those last ten pounds. You are really getting fed up with how slowly the weight is coming off. Despite integrating exercise into your schedule, you are noticing that the weight is taking a long time to budge. You:

   A. Decide to go on a low-carb, high-protein diet and restrict all fattening foods: you are determined to stay on this for several months, and you do, ignoring all tempting foods.

   B. Decide to go on a low-carb, high-protein diet, but then after several weeks start to eat carbs in higher quantities again, spending alternate days bingeing on carbs and then returning to high-protein, no-carb eating.

   C. Decide to really diet but end up cutting back just a little on your food intake, all the while feeling mildly guilty and uncomfortable and wishing you could diet better and be more disciplined.

   D. Decide that the next ten pounds will most likely come off in time as you stop nursing and return to your usual activities. You continue to have a relaxed attitude about your food intake.

What Your Responses Mean

- If most of your answers were As, you are probably quite rigid and used to feeling comfortable with the control you have over food. Controlling your food has quite likely worked for you in the past, but you might have a harder time as your child starts to fight with you over control issues and uses food as a forum for doing this. It is useful to understand your tendency to be controlling because it is possible that your children will detect this trait, especially as they enter the developmental stages in which their main task is to differentiate themselves from you, establish their will, and test their power. At such times, they will most likely use food as an issue or grounds for a fight. It may also be hard for you to figure out how to be less controlling with relation to food.

- If you responded mostly with Bs, you are quite likely a chronic dieter who has spent much of your life alternating between eating excessively and restricting your food. If you eat one food more than you'd planned, you have a hard time forgiving yourself; the only way out is to promise yourself that you will restrict your intake tomorrow. You continue eating in this on-and-off-again manner and may have difficulty dealing with those days when your child has been to a birthday party and then the circus and has eaten mainly cake and ice cream. You may feel that you did a terrible job as a parent by allowing this to happen.

- If you answered mostly with Cs, you, like most of us, live in a culture that bombards us with the idea that we should feel guilty when we are eating dessert and fattening foods, but you remain relatively relaxed when you do indulge in those foods. You can forgive yourself, because you realize that your generally healthy habits will make up for your day of overeating. You may have a relatively easy time if your child has a day of bad eating, but you will be sure to integrate more healthy meals during the week.

- If you answered mostly with Ds, you are probably relaxed about food and diet. You don't really worry much about whether your kids are getting enough nutrition because you trust that you are giving them access to a complete range of foods. You let your children make a lot of their own choices, and it is not stressful for you if they have a day of junk eating.

Rarely do we fall neatly into one category; more often, we float from one to another on the continuum. You may not always be an A or a D, and you may find that you plot yourself somewhere between A and B or between C and D. As you begin to see how flexible or rigid you are—with yourself and your kids—consider this: the more flexible you are able to be, the more likely it is that your children will learn to make good decisions about food.

Overinvolved, Underinvolved, and Unrealistic Standards

In addition to evaluating how flexible or rigid you are, it is also helpful to see how involved you are in your children's eating behavior. Generally parents deal with their children in one of three ways. Again, you will probably fall somewhere along a spectrum rather than at one extreme or another. Once you figure out where you tend to fall, you will be better able to see how you've been dealing with your kids and their eating behavior:

- **Are you overinvolved?**

  Overinvolved parents have a hard time relaxing and not worrying about how their child is eating. They tend to hover and make comments.

- **Are you underinvolved?**

  An underinvolved parent tends to ignore his or her child's eating behavior—whether the child is always asking for a third helping or seems fixated on losing weight. A parent's underinvolvement often stems from a wish not to replicate her or his own parent's overinvolved behavior, or it can be a result of not having developed the tools to deal with these issues.

- **Do you have unrealistic standards for how your children should be eating?**

  A parent who sets unrealistic standards usually does so either because she has set such standards for herself or because she feels guilt and dread at not upholding such standards of "good" eating. Additionally, a parent may have unrealistic ideas about their child's body type, which can, in turn, result in the parent having difficulty accepting that child's natural eating habits.

The Overinvolved Parent

The overinvolved parent usually has not established enough distance between his own food legacy and how he is dealing with his children's eating behavior.

Tom and Nancy are two high-powered lawyers in New York City. They are attractive, bright, and articulate, and both of them are short; he is five six, and she is five two.

They came to see me about their five-year-old son, Alex, who they said had almost always been on the low end of the chart for height and weight. (No surprise to me, given their stature.) They were worried that Alex, who had always been an extraordinarily picky eater, was not getting proper nutrition. As a result, there was a great deal of tension in the home, and it was often difficult for them to eat with other families. "All the other kids eat well enough, but our son barely eats anything," Tom said in exasperation.

Not only did Alex hardly eat at all, but he also often insisted on eating the one food he had picked that week. It might be cheese puffs or peanut butter—the food of the week varied—but he ate only a very small amount and rarely more than one food at a time. Tom and Nancy said they were being pressured by well-meaning friends and relatives to be more strict with Alex. And they also felt stressed by always having to make sure they had Alex's food of the week with them wherever they went. Most important, Tom and Nancy worried that Alex would never get the nutrition he needed, and that he would certainly never learn to eat well.

I asked them what their pediatrician had said in answer to the questions, "Is he on the growth curve? Is he thriving? Does he have energy?" They reassured me that he found Alex to be in perfect health for his size and was not at all worried.

They further described their son as having abundant amounts of energy and told me that he was very involved in sports and hardly ever got sick. We then talked about the foods Alex did eat: while his menu was limited (his diet consisted mainly of soy milk, cheese puffs, peanut butter, ap-

How Do Physicians and Health Care Providers Assess Children's General Health?

ONE IMPORTANT PARAMETER is how they develop according to their own individual growth chart. Dr. Elizabeth Rider, Assistant Professor of Pediatrics at Harvard Medical School, suggests that you "keep track of your child's growth and development as part of regular visits to your pediatrician's office. If your child remains consistent and is growing in height and weight in the proper ratio, this is reassuring for his overall health." She also mentions that some parents are concerned about their children's body types. "Whether your child has a small, medium, or large frame, we consider the child's weight in the context of that frame."

ples, and orange juice), it was clear that he was receiving significant protein, carbohydrates, vitamins, and minerals—all of which are the building blocks of sound nutrition. (You will learn more about specific food requirements in chapter four.) But despite my reassurances that their son was obviously healthy, Tom and Nancy remained concerned and uncomfortable with the fact that Alex ate so little.

I then inquired about their own eating habits as children, asking them if they too had been small kids. Their responses? Yes, they had similar picky eating habits, and yes, they were both small. It quickly became apparent that Tom was very ashamed of how his child ate. When I pressed him a bit, he admitted that Alex reminded him of himself as a child, when he was teased for being small and called "a skinny wimp." Despite all Tom's success as an adult, he still cringed at the idea of his son's being teased and made to feel ashamed, as he had been when he was a child. Additionally, Tom was very sensitive to the judgment of other parents who he thought were being critical of his parenting. Tom felt that they wanted him to simply lay down the law and force Alex to eat the foods that all the other kids were eating. In fact, he had often tried to bully Alex into eating more and admitted that his son ate far less with him than with Nancy.

As we began to work together, it became clear that the first order of business was for both Tom and Nancy to become more comfortable and accepting of both their own food legacies and their issues regarding their son's body type. Once Tom, for example, understood that his son was happy, healthy, and not being teased, he was able to separate Alex's experience from his own past.

If you tend to be overinvolved in your child's eating

Food for Thought

MANY PARENTS HAVE unresolved issues with food. Often simply becoming aware of these attitudes is enough to allow them to begin approaching their kids' eating behaviors more objectively. If you continue to have trouble separating your own food issues from your child's eating behaviors, you might want to consult a therapist or a specialist dealing with food issues.

behavior, you may be turning food into a battleground more often than is necessary. Your concern may be based more on your own food legacy than on your child's actual eating behavior. As a result, you may actually be helping to create a problem when no problem exists. Knowing when to back off and give your child more choice will help take the fight out of food.

As you will see, once parents are able to separate their own food legacies from their children's eating behaviors, they have a much easier time guiding children to eat in a balanced, moderate way from all the food groups—which is one of the goals of teaching your kids to eat for life.

The Underinvolved Parent

This next scenario illustrates the challenge of a parent who is underinvolved. Jan is a thirty-five-year-old mother who laughingly calls herself "the obese mom," which is quite ironic, given that she is diminutive and without an ounce of body fat. When she came to consult with me about her overweight son, she told me that when he was born she read the books, felt confident that a child could never overeat, and she did what the books recommended. She laid out a variety of foods on his tray, feeling certain that he would stop eating when he was full.

Jan had a very demanding job, but she trusted her nanny, and her son seemed to be happy and was developing beautifully. What she did not know, however, was that her nanny was constantly feeding him. When he was in the stroller, there was always a bottle in his mouth, and the nanny, an overweight woman herself, was constantly feeding him chocolate bars and cake, giving him the clear signal that food is love.

Jan's son was very attached to the nanny, connected food with love, and soon became a habitual overeater. Jan told me that while she had noticed he was certainly chubby, she figured he was just a large baby. He was thriving, and it was not until when, at the age of three and a half, his pediatrician stated "this child is obese!" that she decided to take action. "That was my wake-up call," Jan explained.

Despite her reluctance to deprive her child of the caregiver he adored, Jan was constantly fighting with the nanny about the way she was feeding him. Jan had even begun to suspect that the woman, while outwardly agreeing with Jan, was sneaking him food. The difficult part, however, was that Jan too equated food with love; to her, being a good mother was nurturing her child with a lot of food. Her mother had been completely uninvolved with her children's meals, and the kids pretty much fed themselves, mostly relying on junk food. So when Jan became a mother, she was determined never to deprive her child of food and to offer him anything he wanted. Although she worried about her nanny's overfeeding of her child, she also saw this as an expression of the nanny's love and concern and doubted her own ability to set up the structure he would need to break his connection between food and love. (See page 207 for more information on how to deal with babysitters, nannies, and other caregivers.)

She also knew that she needed help from someone who would be able to provide the structure she feared. Her solution was to hire a new nanny, who completely changed the household. This new nanny was outraged by the boy's eating habits and believed strongly that children do not need to eat all day long or to constantly have sippy cups of juice at the park. Her attitude was that a child needed to learn to wait, eat at snack and mealtimes, and certainly eat less sugar.

While her advice made sense to Jan, she still had difficulty with what she saw as depriving her son of his favorite treats. As a result of growing up drinking Coke and eating Twinkies, Jan had never learned much about nutrition or about integrating sweets and treats in a balanced way. And never having had a weight problem, she had never been forced to confront the negative effects of eating such sweet, fatty foods.

In fact, as she eventually came to realize, Jan herself had reinforced her son's food-as-love connection. One of her favorite activities had been making cookies with him, after which they'd both eat the batter and then the cookies. Her son also loved this cozy, warm time when Jan was nurturing herself as well as him.

When her new nanny witnessed this cookie-baking activity, she was outraged: "Why on earth would you choose making cookies when your child is overweight?" This was yet another wake-up call for Jan, to see how clearly her own food legacy was impacting her vision of how to be a good mom.

Following the nanny's lead, she began to set up clear standards with regard to eating and to teach her son about nutrition (see chapter four for more information on this). But it was still a struggle. During the first two weeks, while he was withdrawing from sugar, he had headaches, he was cranky, and he had difficulty sleeping. But once he'd broken his attachment to sugar and sweets, he began to eat a variety of foods. Within a year, he had lost twenty-five pounds and matched his percentile for weight. His physician no longer considered him to be overweight.

Jan not only learned how to set limits with her son but also how to talk to him about food and nutrition in a way that he was able to understand and follow. And she realized that, given some choice about when he could have his treat, her son soon became less demanding and learned to incorporate sugar into a healthy diet. (You will find such instructions in chapter four.)

Interestingly, when I asked Jan whether she would have been more concerned about her child's weight in the early years if her child had been a girl rather than a boy, she said vehemently, "Yes! I would never have allowed my daughter to be overweight like that!" Jan's comment is consistent with a general prejudice in our culture: we tend to be much more concerned about girls (and young women) being overweight than boys (and young men).

If you think you are underinvolved in your child's eating behavior, first assess her nutritional intake. Is she getting enough balance in her diet? Does the pediatrician think she is growing consistently in height and weight? Have you begun teaching your child about nutrition, or are you simply hoping that she will figure it out on her own?

These are just some questions that you can use to help you assess your child's eating behavior, especially if you suspect she may be overeating. Again, in part two, you will learn the four steps of eating for life, which will give you tools and exercises to help you become more positively involved in your child's eating behavior.

The Parent with Unrealistic Standards

Not unlike the overinvolved parents, those with unrealistic standards tend to be more restrictive about the foods they want or will allow their children to eat. They are so focused on controlling their child's food intake that they tend to ignore or overlook the child's particular behavior, stage of development, temperament, or eating style.

When Casey came to meet with me for a few sessions, she was very upset about the fact that her seven-year-old son was beginning to put on some weight. In fact, she had already consulted with her pediatrician, who had reassured her that although he was looking a bit "chunkier" than usual (he'd always been a bit stocky but was also muscular and never had much fat), this was typical of boys who were about to enter a growth spurt. The pediatrician then reminded Casey how to provide good nutrition for her son and help him stay away from junk food.

When I asked why the doctor's response hadn't allayed her fears, Casey said, "I have been feeding Ben the healthiest food you could imagine for his whole life. How could he be gaining weight? It's impossible!"

Casey claimed that she gave Ben a lot of freedom to choose the range of foods he wanted at mealtimes and always prepared healthy foods he could have at his disposal in the fridge and the pantry. Up to that point, things seemed to have been working out just fine. So when he began gaining weight, she became very frustrated.

"Could he be eating junk food when he's at other kids' homes or at school?" I asked.

At first Casey was reluctant to admit such a possibility.

But when she questioned him afterward, she learned that even though he had completely understood her and her husband's feelings about junk food and sugar and had absorbed their attitudes, he had started to eat these foods outside the house. But why hadn't he told his mother? Simply because he knew it would have upset her. And, as a result, he was also showing signs of feeling ashamed about both his sneaking behavior and his weight gain.

I knew that before we could focus on helping Ben manage his weight, we had to address Casey's own attitude toward her son's eating habits and what his "chunkiness" seemed to mean to her. In other words, before she could deal with Ben's weight gain and his desire to eat junk food, she had to admit that her own food legacy was exacerbating the situation. She then told me that she had been raised by an extremely progressive mom who fed her children organic and health foods, emphasizing this way of eating as a way of life. There had never been a bit of junk food or sugar in their house, and Casey had accepted that rule. In fact the rigidity and structure actually appealed to her temperament, and she had been raising Ben the same way. Further, she herself had never had any problem with overeating or weight gain.

I counseled Casey that she needed to get over worrying that she would be a bad mother and become more flexible about junk food and sugar for the time being, because Ben was, in fact, overeating these foods. I advised her to open up and try to be a bit less rigid about allowing some of these foods in their own house. I also encouraged her to allow her son to experiment with these foods within her sight so that he would feel less guilty about eating something that was forbidden.

Casey then came up with her own parameters: she was comfortable with letting Ben have some junk food, but he had to eat healthy food first. She also found another way to reduce her son's need to overeat these foods outside the home: she designated one dinner a week as Silly Supper, when Ben could decide what he wanted to eat, and she was not allowed to comment on it.

I was also helping Casey teach Ben about nutrition. Although she had always fed him the healthiest of foods, she had never thought about teaching him how or why to care for his own body. Once he understood that Casey respected his own feelings about sugar and junk food, even though they were different from hers, Ben was motivated to listen to what she had to say about nutrition. The more information and freedom Casey gave him, the less he overate, and eventually he stopped asking for snacks from other children.

If you think you may be setting unrealistic standards, you need to take a hard look at your rules and parameters.

Establishing Rules and Parameters

IT'S UP TO PARENTS to clearly communicate the food and eating rules of the house so that children know what the limits are. However, it's equally important for parents to allow children some choice and freedom within the scope of their chosen parameters. It's also important for parents to stay flexible and allow the rules to slip occasionally. In chapter eight, you will be able to review and reconsider how you want to establish parameters in your home.

Are they too rigid? Are they causing your child to sneak or hoard food? If so, try to become more familiar with the essentials of nutrition (see chapter four), so that you will feel more comfortable as you ease into giving your child more responsibility for making choices and decisions.

It's also important that you are honest with yourself about your child's unique body type. Is your son small like Alex? Might this be why he tends to eat so little? Is that painful for you to see because you struggled with your own stature as a child and adult? Is your daughter larger than her brother? If so, do you worry that she will not feel comfortable in her body because you yourself struggled with weight as a child? Does your daughter have a larger frame than you? Are you uncomfortable or nervous that she may be big or overweight?

In order to be realistic about your child's genetic inheritance, you must be honest in assessing your own feelings about your child's body. Are you uncomfortable? Ashamed? Worried? Be frank with yourself; these feelings happen. The important thing is to make sure you understand their connection to your own experience so that you can separate your feelings from the way you communicate with your child.

If you think you may be asking your child to live up to unrealistic standards, you may want to consider how your strictness could be contributing to the difficulty your child is having with following your rules. If a child continues to be unable to meet rigid parameters, she will end up feeling like a failure and have little sense of how to take care of her own body. So try and ease up on yourself and your children and build more Silly Suppers into your routine!

Are You Ready for the Next Step?

Separating your own food legacy from your children's eating behaviors is not always easy. It can be challenging to look at yourself in the mirror and see your own food habits and attitudes. Just know that even though you may not resolve your own food issues right away, you can still help your children learn to have a healthy relationship with food, unfettered by negative tape loops. Essentially, once you are able to be clear and objective in dealing with your kids' eating behavior, you will be able to replace your overinvolvement, underinvolvement, or unrealistic standards with a new attitude by doing three things:

- Give up some control.
- Give children some freedom to make their own decisions.
- Observe your children and separate your feelings and behavior from theirs.

These three objectives require you to be flexible about your kids' relationship with food. You need to trust not only your own ability to teach and guide your children but also your children's innate desire and ability to take care of their own bodies.

The minute our children move from breast milk and formula to solid foods, they become very sensitive to the attitudes we parents have toward food. Without our even realizing it, we broadcast our own preferences, dislikes, and hang-ups loudly and clearly to our children, sending them, often unwittingly, messages that can contradict our intentions. By neutralizing such negative interference, you can and will accomplish the three objectives outlined above.

In the next chapter, you will begin to unravel what may be going on with your children and food by looking at them in terms of their developmental stage and temperament. Within this context, you might find that your children's eating behavior, though annoying or frustrating to you, is indeed perfectly normal for their age. And if you still want to help them change their behavior, you will also find helpful tips on how to make suggestions that are age appropriate.

CHAPTER TWO

Factor In Your Child's Developmental Stage

I thought I'd never see the day when my daughter started to like her veggies again! She stopped eating them at age one and a half and suddenly when she just turned seven, she asked me for some green beans!

MOTHER OF TWO, NEW YORK CITY

WHEN IT COMES TO FEEDING our children and teaching them how to eat for life, their developmental stage—physically, intellectually (that is, cognitively), emotionally, and psychologically—plays a big role in how we react and respond to their eating habits. When our children are infants, we tend to be much more in tune with how they are growing and developing. We are looking for their developmental milestones, such as their first smile, their first clasp of a spoon, even their first temper tantrum. Once they move beyond the age of two, however, and our visits to the pediatrician become less frequent, we tend to think less about exactly where our kids are developmentally and more about their behavior—at home, in school, and so on. What we need to be aware of is the fact that the way our child behaves around food may have much more to do with his being three or six years old than with any deeper, more complicated behavioral issue. Therefore, the more information you have about child development, the more perspective and insight you will have on what might be going on inside your kid's fast-maturing brain.

Debra is a vibrant, petite brunette mother whom I met at one of my lectures. When she subsequently came to see me in my office, she was worried about her young daughter Natalie, who had been a "great eater" during her first year. When Natalie moved from breast milk to solid foods, Debra was delighted to see that she loved to feed herself, picking up pieces of fruit, chicken, even small bits of boiled potato. In fact every mother in her playgroup envied Debra because Natalie was eating so well. "What a great eater she is!" they'd tell Debra. "I wish my son were as enthusiastic about his food!" Then suddenly, when Natalie reached twelve months, she began to reject all her favorite foods. "She used to love yogurt, green veggies, and other baby foods. Now all she's interested in is her bottle! And just when am I supposed to take her bottle away and give her a sippy cup?" Debra was distraught.

I explained to Debra that Natalie's turning twelve months was a huge factor in her sudden dismissal of foods she had previously eaten without contest. Like most one-year-olds, she had begun testing her ability to impact the world around her through the cause and effect of her actions: "If I throw the ball, it hits the floor. If I push this toy, the sound comes out." I tried to reassure Debra that her daughter's response was not only age appropriate but also completely healthy developmentally. One-year-olds are so excited by their improved motor skills, their ability to walk (or striving to do so), and the fact that they can accomplish such tasks by themselves, that they are often too absorbed to bother eating. A whole new world is opening up to them, and they don't necessarily want to spend a lot of time picking up food, putting it in their mouths, or chewing! If they can drink a bottle and move on to their next interest, pushing that ball around, or toddling over to that window, well, certainly that is their preferred choice. And yet, it is unsettling for parents to observe a baby who was previously an adventurous and excited eater suddenly lose interest in food.

I suggested that Debra try to zero in on when Natalie was just hungry enough to be interested, but not so starved that she wanted only her bottle. I also suggested that she pace Natalie, placing small amounts of food on her tray and watching for Natalie's signs of hunger and fullness. Debra learned not to rush and try to feed Natalie one hour after she had eaten if she didn't show any sign of hunger. I also suggested that she keep in mind how rested or tired Natalie might be. If she seemed to have energy to burn, then let her burn it and wait until she lost some steam before introducing food again. After Debra played around with the timing and began to see that Natalie did indeed sit down and show renewed interest in the foods she used to eat, Debra began to breathe a sigh of relief.

Once they've identified the typical behaviors of their child's developmental stage, parents are better able to take their pediatrician's advice and relax. This chapter, then, offers a general description of the various developmental stages children go through from nine months through age nine and explains how the particular stage they are experiencing intersects with and affects their eating behaviors. I've delineated this age range because most eating issues begin or become noticeable when children have been introduced to solid foods, and after the age of nine, when children enter either prepuberty or puberty itself, their relationship with food becomes more complicated because of radical changes in hormones and body chemistry.

Now let's take a look at developmentally appropriate behaviors for the various age groups.

Cluing In to Developmentally Appropriate Behavior

In the years since Erik Erikson first pioneered the study of child development, many other theorists and clinicians have contributed to our understanding of how children grow. Indeed, we know that growth is always multidimensional, ongoing, and occurs in fits and starts. Erikson codified his ideas of child development into eight phases or stages, each one of which presents the child (and later the teenager and adult) with a "psychosocial crisis" that demands resolution before the next stage can be navigated satisfactorily. Other thinkers such as Dr. Arnold Gesell, founder of the Gesell Institute of Human Development, and Dr. T. Berry Brazelton focused more on the moments or time periods just before a child makes a developmental breakthrough. Gesell identified developmental stages as occurring between periods of equilibrium. "The good, solid equilibrium of any early age seems to need to break up into *disequilibrium* before the child can reach a higher or more mature stage of equilibrium, which again will be followed by disequilibrium" (4–5). Brazelton takes a slightly different approach, using the concept of "touchpoints," universal indications of "predictable times that occur just before a surge of rapid growth in any line of development—motor, cognitive, or emotional—when, for a short time, the child's behavior falls apart" (xi). At such times, he says, children often regress or act out, showing that they are either afraid, frustrated, or unsure of moving forward.

A simple way to think of developmental touchpoints is in terms of the old adage "Three steps forward, one step back." As a child is moving forward in one area of development (for example, learning to walk and feed himself), he regresses in another area (cries more intensely when his mother leaves the room). For example, a five-year-old child might display regression in another way. If he is in the midst of striving for independence and individuation, demonstrated by his new interest in riding his bike down to the end of his street, he might show other signs of regression, such as once again clinging tightly to his favorite stuffed animal or blanket in order to help himself fall asleep at night.

Not surprisingly, some children may choose food as the forum for expressing their disequilibrium and may exhibit changes in behavior that you as a parent do not expect. For example, your child might suddenly "hate" his favorite food, throw a fit when you feed him what he always loved, or just plain make a change in his behavior with relation to food. If this happens, what you need to keep in mind is that these sudden changes may have little to do with the food itself and much more to do with the developmental changes your child is experiencing.

It's also important to keep in mind that children develop at different rates—cognitively, emotionally, and physically. Parents of more than one child are all too familiar with this fact. As Charlene said, "Of my four children, Brian, my youngest, developed his motor skills way before the other three children, but he lagged behind in speech." Children have their own genetic imprint for when they will develop their skills, and this rate of development can impact their eating behavior. How children's senses develop, for example, has a particular effect. The senses, of course, include sight, sound, touch, taste, and smell. The last three in particular— the senses of touch (texture), taste, and smell—and their unique pace of development are going to have a direct impact on children's behavior with food. How the brain processes, organizes, and interprets this sensory information is called sensory integration. One child is an early talker, the other an early walker. One reads by the age of three, the other begins to read in first grade. These are all variations of what is considered to be normal, and the same is true of how and when children develop and integrate their senses.

Helaine Ciporin, C.S.W., a learning specialist with an expertise in the area of sensory integration, puts it very well: "What we need to understand is senses develop slowly and get more refined as you age. For instance, vision: babies are born seeing shadows and their vision gradually gets more and more refined as the muscles in their eyes develop to the point where, generally, by the age of seven their eye muscles can hold the letter that they see steady enough that they can begin to read. Each sense goes from the gross to the refined at its own pace."

The wide variation we see in the age when children begin

to read is therefore closely related to the rate at which their vision develops. If we can begin to see how the development of their other senses may impact the way they eat, we can begin to let ourselves off the hook and truly see why we need not take it personally when one two-year-old is a very picky eater while another eats everything her mother offers! Following is a guide that describes how your child's stage of development often intersects with his eating behaviors. This information offers general guidelines rather than rules written in stone. It may, however, save you when you watch in horror as your toddler flings a bowl of peas across the room!

Ages Nine to Eighteen Months

At this age, infants are beginning to acquire more advanced motor skills as they also experience the first stages of emotional separation from their primary caregiver, usually the mother. These increased motor skills are what often prompt the separation anxiety: the more they become independent of the parent, the more they begin to feel they want to make sure the parent is still there.

At the same time, they have begun to move from breast milk or formula to more solid foods. Children at this age start experimenting with new foods as parents present a wider range of options. Cognitively, the child's interest in food is more about the experience of eating than it is about the food itself. Parents will observe children attempting to self-feed and playing with food. As they near the end of this stage and become more mobile—able to crawl or walk—their interest in eating and food begins to wane, particularly as they become excited about exploring the world.

Keeping a Food Journal

WHEN PARENTS BECOME more aware of exactly what their children have eaten, they often worry less about their eating enough. The main technique I advise parents to use is keeping a food journal. This can be any kind of record in which you write down the amount and the frequency of what your child eats—from meals to numbers of bottles to snacks.

Some children even start to thin out, losing some of their baby fat. As a result, this is a time when some parents begin to worry that their child isn't getting enough to eat. As one mother said, "My daughter is almost sixteen months and she barely eats anything! How is she going to grow?" I always ask parents to try to make note of what the child is actually eating—it can appear that she hardly eats at all when in fact she eats very little at any one time but eats continually throughout the day.

This is also the stage at which parents worry that too little eating might interfere with sleep patterns. They are concerned that if their child doesn't eat "enough" during the day he will wake up hungry in the middle of the night and need to eat. (See page 124 for more information on addressing this issue.)

Keep in Mind

- Kids of this age group need far less food than we think.
- Little bits of food add up.

- They often lose interest in food.

- They do not need to eat at night, even if they have eaten very little during the day. Their bodies will adjust the next day.

- They don't sit still for meals very long.

- They will rely more on bottles or sippy cups if you give these to them and will eat fewer solids. Make sure you do not give them too much juice—stick with water, and have them get more of their nutrition through foods. Milk and soy milk are also good, but if you rely too heavily on milk, your child is likely to fill up and not want to eat.

- Try to help your children learn that eating happens at specific times by not overfeeding them with snacks. Think of what you load up the stroller with when you go to the park. If they whine for snacks but tend to eat very little at mealtimes, try to distract them from snacks. Setting limits and saying no is not very effective at this age. Distraction works best!

- Make snacks as nutrient rich as possible. That way, if your child seems to prefer grazing to eating full meals, you will worry less about her nutrition.

- If your child refuses to eat, don't force the issue. You can leave the food out for him and reintroduce it an hour later when he may be hungrier. After that, you have the right to stop offering food, and your child will eventually get the message when you say: "Last chance!" (This rule applies to all ages—see ahead!)

Ages Eighteen Months to Three Years

During this stage children are moving out of infancy into toddlerhood. Once they begin to walk, they become very interested in exploring their expanding environment. They become more sure on their feet and better able to walk, run, and climb. And when these motor skills improve, children also begin to explore separation from their caregivers.

At the beginning of this stage, from ages one and a half to two, children are often less adventurous with food. They tend to eat only when hungry, and parents often describe their children as never eating a "full meal" but rather "grazing" throughout the day. This eating style can be a struggle for parents who think children should eat three square meals a day in order to be and stay healthy. But, as you will see in chapter four, children actually need much less food than most of us think, and they usually get plenty of nutrients in whatever it is they do eat. Again, try to make their snacks as nutrient rich as possible.

Snack Rules

MY GENERAL APPROACH to snacks is as follows:

- The younger the child, the more likely she needs snacks between meals.
- Make these snacks as nutrient rich as possible.
- If your child tends to rely on snacks throughout the day, think of snacks as minimeals, offering something substantive, such as a piece of pizza, a hot dog, or a chicken nugget.

In the middle of this stage, around two and a half years old, many children begin to express their desire to separate and individuate from their parent or caregiver by asserting their will—hence what we often refer to as the "terrible twos." And this same interest in testing their will can also be played out around food. They want to do more for themselves, including feeding, which often means getting a lot on the floor.

This stage is also characterized by greatly increased language ability, with children jumping from fifty to more than five hundred words in a few short years. However, although children can now understand much of what their parents say, they are typically not as good at expressing their own wishes, which can cause them to become very frustrated. Some of this frustration begins to play out around food—for example, in their insistence on eating some foods but not others or in their suddenly refusing to eat what had been one of their favorite foods. I hear many parents say that between the ages two and three their children begin to refuse vegetables. Michael Traister, M.D., a pediatrician in New York City, says on the topic: "It's very typical of toddlers to refuse vegetables because their colors and textures seem exotic. Toddlers tend to prefer foods that are bland in color and texture."

My advice to parents at this stage is to approach eating as a fun activity and not to worry too much about their child's appetite, which can seem small and come in spurts.

Keep in Mind

- If she starts to refuse veggies, don't worry. You can rely more on fruits, or let her find one fruit she might eat. If she won't eat fruit you can always offer her vitamins to make yourself more comfortable—but don't sweat it!

- Kids this age can begin to use food, like clothing, as a way to express their preferences and their differences from you, and this is just the beginning! If they refuse to eat, do not force the issue. Toward the end of this age span, kids will also begin to use food to test you. Resist joining the fight!

- Children may eat very little on some days and then fill up on others. Do not let this alarm you. Don't force the food; help them track their hunger and respect their fullness.

- Children can also want to eat small amounts all day long. As you are beginning to establish regular meal-times and may not want to travel around with a back-pack full of food, try to distract them when they start whining for a sippy cup. Give them water instead of juice or milk, and get them in the habit of eating a bit less frequently and more at one time. You can do this gradually; stretch the time between feedings from half an hour to an hour to two hours. Be realistic however; this age group may need to eat smaller amounts and therefore may not be able to go without a small snack for as long as older children can.

- If the child has an older sibling, she will have been exposed to sugar and so may start demanding it: determine the parameters you are comfortable with, but give your child some choice.

- At this stage, children start to want to control their food as a way to assert control on their environment. If they have begun to demand certain foods such as desserts or sweets, try to distract them. If the distraction doesn't work and the child returns to his request for the food, let him have it, knowing that, nine times out of ten, children will quickly forget the fight and move on to another activity. (See pages 61–65 for more information and advice about dealing with the Food Demander eating style.)

Ages Three to Five Years

This stage is characterized predominantly by children's wanting to establish even more separateness, independence, and power—developments that are played out with (or against) their parents. This often results in struggles between children and parents concerning guidelines about food, especially with reference to sugar. During this stage, every food interaction between you and your child can feel like a negotiation, with the child seemingly pushing the limit and asking herself, "How can I be the boss?" For this reason, parents need to be clear on their guidelines and stick firmly to them. At the same time, however, parents need to extend some control to children as a way of acknowledging their intense need for separateness. Two easy ways to give some control without relinquishing your firm guidelines is to let your child establish how hungry she is and offer her a couple of choices about either what or when to eat. If, for example, she says she is "done" eating, then don't argue and try to make her finish what's on her plate. It is crucial that you consistently support her need for independence so that she is able to build confidence in herself.

Keep in Mind

- You need to continue to set parameters that are comfortable for you but not too rigid.

- Give your children choices within these parameters. For example, let them choose when they can have their treat—such as after lunch or after dinner.

- Some children will vehemently refuse whatever you make for dinner. You can either insist they eat what's being served or create another option you know the child likes. The alternative should be something that is easy for you to prepare, something you can pull from the cupboard or refrigerator, or something your child can get for herself from the fridge. Children love that independence. And if you do decide that the rule in your house is only one option per night, you can take comfort in the fact that your child will not starve if he goes to bed without supper.

- Children in this age range change their likes and dislikes from week to week, so breathe deeply and always have one or two backup foods they tend to like. If all else fails, offer them cereal for dinner. Do not drive yourself crazy! And do not allow yourself to be held hostage in the kitchen.

- Kids can also use food to create power struggles and to test you. Once you allow them some freedom and choices, these power struggles often dissipate.

- If your child continues to refuse all the options you offer, including foods he has always liked in the past, simply say, "Then you must not be hungry; when you are, we can think about what your body might be telling you it wants to eat." Then leave the room and disengage. Children are eager to engage your attention in this struggle.

- If your child agrees when you suggest he isn't hungry, ask him to sit at the dinner table anyway. He still wants the attention and engagement with you. Then, after a while, you can gently ask him to see if his tummy might be hungry now.

- Children this age can begin to have trouble knowing when to stop eating. Often, this is because they're having trouble moving from eating to the next activity. Encourage them to stop after eating a reasonable amount, and reassure them that they can have more in twenty minutes. Teach them that their stomach needs time to tell their brain whether they are full. (See chapter five, "Step Two: Reboot the Connection Between the Belly and the Head.")

- If you notice that your child consistently cannot seem to stop eating, do the above and engage her in another activity with you. Begin to teach her about listening to her body's signals of fullness and hunger. (See pages 124–28 for specific directions on this.)

- Kids in this age group are also in school, and their social interactions can become more complex. Feelings get hurt. One day is terrific, the next day is terrible. Help your child to notice if he is using food, or more specifically treats, to soothe hurt feelings. (See chapter six about helping your child to separate feelings of hunger from other emotions.)

Ages Five to Seven Years

At this stage of development, children begin to be more conscious and feel prouder of their individual accomplishments. And yet at the same time, children of five going on six are in a natural state of transition. As Dr. Louise Bates-Ames says, "The five-and-a-half-year-old is characteristically hesitant, dawdling, indecisive, or, at the opposite extreme, overdemanding and explosive." As much as they cling to Mother, they are also continuing to separate and grow autonomous. They're gaining a sense of their responsibilities—at school, within the family setting, and with their peers. And by the time children turn six, this transition from one extreme to another can become more internalized. They often feel ambivalent, and decision making becomes difficult or overwhelming. This age group can sometimes eat all day long, but for the most part, their change in eating behavior is a sign of an impending growth spurt and is not, therefore, a cause for concern. Depending on the child's size and rate of growth, parents should also expect variations in appetite.

At times parents will also notice a dramatic shift in tastes, with a child loving peanut butter one week and hating it the next. Keep in mind that children in this age range will continue to test limits around the guidelines you set, particularly when they enter school, begin having playdates, and are more exposed to different families and styles. Very immersed in the routine of school, they are now also becoming increasingly independent of Mother and the home. As a result, you might see your child engaging in a kind of push-pull behavior, at one moment wanting to show you "I can do this all by myself and I know what is good for me," and then regressing into asking for help with something he'd easily been doing for himself.

Keep in Mind

- Children in this age group develop more interest in and have a greater ability to cook or prepare their own meals. Take them grocery shopping and involve them in meal planning; the more responsibility and input they have, the more motivated they will be to take good care of their bodies and the less inclined they are to struggle with you about food.

- They may begin to use food to distract themselves from emotional states such as boredom, sadness, or loneliness. It may be more difficult for them to express themselves in words, but you can help them to identify what they are feeling. (See page 146 for advice on helping kids identify their feelings.)

- They may continue to demand sugar and junk food; again, give them choices. Give them more responsibility and continue teaching in accordance with their growing cognitive ability to take in nutritional information. Be sure to connect this information to the activities they enjoy. (See chapter four for further guidelines.)

- Continue to reinforce rules about eating when they're hungry and stopping when they're full. Help them to connect to their feelings of hunger and fullness if they do not appear to be self-regulating. (See pages 124–28 for the Hunger-Fullness scale and other guidelines.).

- Understand that their food preferences will change dramatically from one week to the next. Be patient and set

Quick Kid-Friendly Options

HERE ARE SOME of the quick, easy, and nutritious alternatives that have been suggested by parents and clients.

- Frozen pizza (Ian's makes a fabulous organic pizza that is low in fat!)
- Hot dogs and vegetarian hot dogs
- Cheese sandwich on grain bread or toast
- Peanut butter and jelly sandwich on grain bread or toast
- Melted cheese in a whole wheat tortilla

limits; offer the meal and have some other choices on hand for them to make or take for themselves so that you are not a slave to the kitchen.

- Know that their level of maturity will ebb and flow. One minute children are pushing for independence, fighting you for food choices and rights; the next minute, they want you to tell them what to do.
- At this stage, they will start to notice what other kids eat, and they might eat other kids' lunches at school. Be careful not to set unrealistic standards for how healthy and nutritious each meal needs to be. If you have none of a certain food (such as sugar and cookies) at home, your children will surely eat more of it at other kids' houses. Try to be flexible as their exposure to the outside world challenges your control, but continue to help them connect to signals of fullness and reinforce

the wisdom of filling up on nutritious foods first and eating dessert for fun.

Ages Seven to Nine Years

An eight-year-old is very different from a seven-year-old. As Dr. Louise Bates-Ames remarks, age seven "stands out, coming as it does between the positive vigor of six and the broad expansiveness of eight." The typical seven-year-old shows a certain tendency toward "withdrawal, of pulling in, of calming down," says Ames. Whereas the six-year-old often relies on his parent to fix certain problems or make certain decisions, "seven expresses a fine new sense of growing independence, a wish at least to try to work things out without help instead of expecting others to solve his problems for him."

Children in this age range sometimes gain weight, particularly if they are prepubescent girls. Parents need to understand that this is usually temporary and try not to worry too much about it.

Since children are becoming more thoughtful and better able to integrate information at this age, it's a good time for parents to reinforce teachings about nutrition and how to take care of their bodies. As a rule children will enjoy that responsibility. Therefore, this is also a great stage for parents to allow their children more freedom to choose their own foods and to be more flexible in their responses to such questions as, "Mom, can I have this cookie?" With their increased intellectual maturity, children in this age range have an easier time reasoning and being reflective, which means they are better able to make thoughtful decisions and connect their choices to potential consequences.

Keep in Mind

- At this age kids, especially girls, can start to look chubby as they gain some weight before puberty sets in. Continue to reinforce the idea of filling up on healthy foods, and using dessert for fun and enjoyment.

- Girls may start wanting to diet. Body consciousness can begin as early as seven, eight, or nine years old. Educate your child about how to eat moderately, teach her not to deprive herself of the foods she loves, and teach her to stay connected to her signals of hunger and fullness. (See pages 124–28 for exercises that will help you do this.)

- At this stage, overeating can start to become a habit if children have difficulty separating hunger from other emotions. Help your children identify their emotions so they don't eat when they're feeling bored, restless, distracted, sad, or anxious. (See pages 146–50 for exercises that will help you do this.)

- Children in this age group continue to wish for independence and responsibility. Capitalize on this by giving them responsibility for taking good care of their bodies; it is their job. Reinforce how well they're doing and be careful not to be critical or judgmental. Encourage their own self-reflection. When they say, "Mom, can I have this chocolate bar?" respond with, "What do you think? What has your body had today? Do you want it now or later? You think about it." If you have educated them properly, as you encourage them to make decisions, they will invariably think of taking good care of their bodies. Respect their decision. This will allow them to feel that you respect how they are caring for themselves.

All children will inevitably move from one developmental stage to the next, yet not always at the same pace or with the same degree of ease or difficulty. As you will see in the next chapter, temperament and personality also play a large, idiosyncratic part in how children behave with relation to food. Indeed, the six eating styles you will meet in the following chapter present another context from which to view your child's behavior. As you become more and more attuned to your individual child's stage of development and eating style, you will feel more comfortable establishing limits, guidelines, and rules for her to follow. You may not yet know exactly what those guidelines are, but I am confident that as you gather more and more information about her and about nutritional recommendations, you will have the clarity and peace of mind to know that you are indeed taking the fight out of food and teaching your child how to eat for life.

CHAPTER THREE

Identify Your Child's Eating Style

One of my sons eats anything I put before him—from sushi to tofu. He's a total adventurer when it comes to food. My other son is so picky he won't touch any food that has a strong color, texture, or smell. They couldn't be more different from one another!

MOTHER OF TWO BOYS, SIX AND EIGHT

DOES YOUR CHILD eat only white or beige food? Does she seem to graze all day, rarely sitting down to eat what you would call a "whole" meal? Or is your child the type who seems to eat nothing for days and then consumes three plates full of his favorite food? Over the years, as I've worked with kids and their parents, I've observed that children demonstrate six distinctive styles of eating that correlate to individual temperament traits. What is a temperament trait? Although we often use this concept loosely, a temperament trait is a genetically determined personality characteristic that both defines and describes the way an individual reacts to the world around him. When we say, for example, "He is so intense and demanding," we are usually referring to the temperament trait intensity of reaction; when we say a child is easily distracted, we are referring to the temperament trait distractibility; and when we say a child is overly sensitive, we are also referring to the temperament trait related to sensory threshold or degree of sensitivity. While these traits can and do change in response to life experiences and environment, they also remain biologically driven. For our purposes, it's useful for parents to know how such characteristics affect their child's eating behavior. Indeed, the six eating styles described in this chapter incorporate those temperament traits that affect eating behavior in kids.

The Six Basic Eating Styles

- *The Food Demander* makes incessant demands for a certain food (usually sweet) or keeps demanding more food. He tends to be temperamentally intense and strong-willed (as opposed to easygoing and compliant) and can end up using food for emotional purposes.

- *The Trouble Transitioner* has trouble either moving from a previous activity to the dinner table or has trouble stopping once he begins eating. He can be very intense and focused and can require a bit more help moving from one activity to the next. Basically, this type of child is highly reactive to change and needs a bit more help adapting to a new situation.

- *The Picky Eater* finds very little he or she likes and keeps changing her mind about the foods she will consent to eat. Kids in this category may, for example, love peanut butter one week and loathe it the next. She may eat only favorite foods. The Picky Eater can be sensitive not only to the colors, smells, and textures of food, but also to other aspects of her environment.

- *The Beige Food Eater* insists on eating foods that are white or beige colored because these foods also tend to be bland in taste. Again, this child can be temperamentally sensitive to his environment and will therefore try to manage this sensitivity by controlling his food choices by color or taste.

- *The Spurt Eater* barely eats for days and then chows down. He will show less interest in food than the more adventurous eater, and it may appear that he subsists on air, only to eat voraciously several days later, playing catch-up with his biological needs.

- *The Grazer* loves to nibble throughout the day and avoids sitting down to a complete meal. This type of eater might be more than usually distracted by outside stimuli and easily engaged in activities other than eating. He might have trouble sitting down to a meal that requires too much of his time and attention. He is off and running, more interested in things other than eating to satisfy his hunger.

Although no doubt annoying at times, these styles are not necessarily harmful, or good or bad. As any parent of more than one child knows, every kid is unique. Some kids are more intense, others have more trouble with change. Use these eating styles as guidelines to make your life easier. The more aware you are of your kids' eating styles, the more understanding and accepting you will be of their—

shall we say—idiosyncrasies. Another important note: your child could easily move from one style to another. These categories are not rigid or set in stone. Since children continue to change, it is important not to fall into the trap of thinking, "Oh this is what my child is like and how she will be forever!"

Look at these eating styles in the context of your child's individual stage of development. For example, at times it can be developmentally appropriate for a toddler who is excited by his expanding world to shift from being an adventurous eater to barely eating at all. Is this child suddenly developing a "problem"? No. He may simply be a Spurt Eater for several months as he gets used to his new motor skills and explores the world around him.

The same goes for the six-year-old who is just beginning to try to make his own choices but who sometimes wants his mother to make decisions for him. As you saw in the previous chapter, a child in this developmental stage is sometimes focused and intense, and tends to be a Food Demander. His wanting more, more, more may, in fact, be a sign of his new intensity and not a real desire for more food. So again, try not to label your child in a concrete or fixed manner but use the six categories as reference points for helping you to detect, prevent, and/or solve any eating problems that may develop. As you observe your child's eating habits, you will begin to identify her eating style, which will help you to find or implement the most appropriate solution. Or you may come to realize that your child does not really have a problem at all but is simply doing what comes naturally for her temperament and stage of development. Indeed, I call these traits eating "styles" because they are not necessarily problems.

The Food Demander

The Food Demander is often strong-willed, intense, and sometimes dramatic. These qualities, while wonderful in some ways, can also be challenging when you want him to follow the rules. Food Demanders want to make their own choices and test the limits of their power. By age three, such children tend to push for sweets *if* they sense there are limits to how much they're allowed.

Lily complained to me that her three-and-a-half-year-old son, Roger, who was ordinarily an adventurous and easygoing eater, had become a tyrant at the dinner table, demanding dessert before the meal even began. Not only was his behavior really getting to her, she said, but she and her husband had begun arguing about how she was handling it.

Roger had a strong need to feel that he had some measure of control, which meant that he also required strong limits. I advised Lily that the first thing she and her husband needed to do was to determine their individual comfort levels and the rules they wanted to establish with regard to mealtimes. They also had to decide how they felt about sugar. In other words, how comfortable did they feel about their son's having one or two desserts?

Lily didn't feel strongly one way or the other, and she certainly did not want to fight too much about it. But her husband, who had grown up eating a very restricted diet consisting primarily of healthful foods, was very opposed to "giving in" to their son, and he often accused Lily of being "too easy." (In chapter eight you will learn more specifically about how to manage partner differences.) Ironically, Lily noticed that their son demanded more cookies when he was with his father than with her.

I recommended that the couple decide on a particular portion size of sugar their son would be allowed to eat, and they agreed upon one dessert a day. Their next step was to explain nutrition to Roger in a way that a three-and-a-half-year-old could understand, such as by talking about the foods that would help build the muscles he needed to climb structures at his new school, or the bones he needed to grow so he would fit into his new roller skates. By engaging the boy's active mind in the process and giving him some of the responsibility, they were able to reinforce the idea that Roger was the "expert" on his own body, and it was, therefore, his job to feed and care for it. Once he understood that they respected his ability to make choices, Lily and her husband introduced the idea that sugar was fun food and important too, but that it didn't fuel Roger's body in the same way as other foods did. Using an analogy suited to Roger's interests, his parents compared the fuel his toy cars needed to run to the fuel his body required. (You can adapt analogies to whatever your child is most passionate about at the moment.)

Lily and her husband then introduced the rule that Roger could have one dessert or treat a day, and it was up to him to decide when to have it. The first day, Roger decided to have his treat with breakfast. His parents agreed but reminded him that having dessert at breakfast meant not being able to have one after dinner.

Later that evening, when Roger asked for his dessert after dinner, he whined and complained, but his parents remained firm, reminding him that it had been his choice to have it at breakfast and that he could make a different choice the next day. And, sure enough, the following day, Roger decided to eat his dessert after dinner, showing that he understood the consequences of his decision. The most difficult part of this entire exercise was for Lily to resist giving in when he put up a fuss. Within several days, Roger was more engaged in the process, felt proud of himself for being in charge of his decisions, and stopped persisting in his demands.

Of course, every day did not go perfectly, and at times Roger would fall back into his demanding behavior, but now his parents had a clearer framework within which to work, and they felt much more comfortable with their ability to handle Roger's "tyrannical" attitude (which was fairly typical of his stage of development, yet exacerbated by his willful temperament). They had to laugh to themselves when, just a year later, they overheard Roger saying to his cousin, "You're not really going to eat all that candy, are you? You need to feed your body healthy food!" (This was after a birthday party when they noticed that, in fact, he had eaten some candy and put away the rest to save for the next day and week, as he put it.) Lily and her husband are happy to report that Roger has also returned to being more adventurous with food, and that mealtimes are no longer a power struggle.

Tips for Dealing with Food Demanders

- Come up with one or two easy options from which your children can choose if they don't like what you have prepared for dinner. Yogurt, cereal, or a piece of fruit are things kids often choose. But don't worry if they don't eat. If they are hungry, they will eat more tomorrow.

- Since Food Demanders often insist on sugar or junk food, educate them about the fact that though these foods may taste good, they don't provide their bodies with fuel. (See more about dealing with junk food and sugar on pages 106–16).

- Establish clear rules about treats such as soda, junk food, and sweets. You may want to give your child some control by letting him decide when he can have his treat, but you control how much he gets and how often he gets it.

- Continue to reinforce your child's choices: does she want the cookie tomorrow as soon as she wakes up or would she rather wait until after dinner?

Some Advice for Handling the Very Intense Child

- Emphasize to the child that more food is available, but it may take a bit of time for his belly to signal to his brain that he is full.
- Suggest doing another activity together to help him calm down.
- If he continues to demand more and more food, reassure him that he can have more if he is still hungry.

- Try not to say NO as a reflex. The Food Demander will only take that response as fodder for a fight.
- If you give in every once in a while, it is not the end of the world. Consistency need not be 100 percent absolute. Remind yourself that your child will eat more nutritiously tomorrow. You are still in charge; you are just choosing to make your life easier at that moment.

The Trouble Transitioner

The child who fits into this category has difficulty moving from one activity to the next. He may, therefore, have trouble starting to eat or stopping once he has started. These are the children who put up a fuss and often say they're not hungry when you ask them to sit down at the dinner table. Or, conversely, after finishing one bowl of ice cream, they may want one more. After two giant slices of pizza, they'll say they're "starving." Trouble Transitioners can also get very focused on the tastes and sensations of the food and have difficulty transitioning from this stimulation, which can result in chronic overeating.

Stacey came to me for help because her seven-year-old daughter, Courtney, had begun to gain weight. Stacey was uncomfortable with the change in her daughter's appearance and her husband's apparent lack of concern about the issue. Stacey was a woman who had not struggled much with weight and who took pride in her fit body. But because her own mother was quite overweight, Stacey feared that Courtney would become like her grandmother. Although Stacey admitted she felt ashamed about her need and wish for her daughter to be thin and attractive, she also admitted that she was growing increasingly uncomfortable as Courtney was becoming larger than most of the other girls at her school.

In the past, Stacey had given Courtney a lot of freedom to choose the foods she wanted and had always believed that exposing her daughter to a range of foods with little or no restriction was the "healthiest" approach to use. But when she began to insist on more and more dessert, and then began to gain weight and change shape, Stacey started to worry that her hands-off approach might not be working.

First, Stacey and I discussed all Stacey's own issues with relation to food. It turned out that because of her reluctance to restrict her daughter's food she had not noticed that she actually needed a bit more structure. When it finally became clear that Courtney continued to ask for more food, even after having had second helpings, Stacey began to figure out that her daughter must be needing something else. The question was, What did she need? And how was Stacey supposed to handle the situation without communicating that Courtney didn't know how she felt if she was saying she wanted more food?

I suggested that Stacey use the following steps to help her daughter figure out if she was really still hungry, or if she really needed help transitioning from the activity of eating. Eating can be very stimulating. It takes the focus off everything else, and if a child enjoys eating, he or she may have difficulty shifting gears—what I call decelerating—and may, at times, need help making transitions. The key here is to help the child know that if she is truly hungry, she can absolutely eat. Many kids like Courtney, who are Trouble Transitioners, begin to lose their innate connection to their bodies as they become focused on the stimulation of the food in their mouth and they do not stop long enough to pay attention to the more subtle sensation in their stomach telling them they are full. This can lead to chronic overeating and a need to reset their satiety signal. (See Step Two, chapter five, for additional help in dealing with this issue.)

While some kids don't want to stop eating, others go to the opposite extreme and won't go near a meal until they are practically starving because their trouble with transitions prevents them from paying attention to their bodies' hunger signals. One mother of a seven-year-old boy came to me asking for help regarding her son's refusal to come to the table and eat with the family. "He always puts up a fight. It takes him forever to sit down and eat. What should I do?" she asked. I explained that although there could be several possible reasons for her son's refusal to come to the table, more than likely he was having trouble transitioning from one activity to another. I suggested that she and her husband give him some tools to help him make the transition less stressful, such as signaling him that dinner would be ready in thirty minutes, then fifteen, and finally five.

Once his parents began to incorporate this strategy, their son gradually came to accept the rule that he come to the table and sit with the rest of the family during dinner. If he didn't want to eat what was offered, he had to acknowledge this to his mother instead of flat out refusing or pushing his plate away. He learned that it was okay if he didn't like a particular dish, but he had to take responsibility for what he was going to eat. The easier it became for the boy to make the transition, the less conflict there was at the dinner table—for everyone.

Another way to make the transition less stressful would be to institute a very structured activity for the half hour before mealtime. This might be doing homework or setting the table, or some other activity that shifts a child's attention to the kitchen and meal preparation.

Tips for Dealing with Trouble Transitioners

- If your child has trouble knowing when to stop eating, tell him he needs to wait ten minutes because his brain may not yet have gotten the message that he is full.

- Make sure the child knows that if she is still hungry when she checks in with her body, of course she can eat more. Also, it's very important to respect your child's food choices; if she says she wants pizza, let her have pizza. Don't suggest an apple just because you think it's better for her. This is an instance where it's important to give your children some control so that you enable them to reap the benefits of the lesson at hand: how to tap into and pay attention to their hunger signals.

- If after twenty minutes, she has not asked for food and has continued with her new activity, you will have taught her a valuable lesson about paying attention to her own signals of hunger and fullness.

- Since Trouble Transitioners need your attention and help shifting gears, suggest an activity they can do with you: help you clear the table, wash the dishes, chat over a glass of water or a cup of tea, play a game, or read a book.

It's up to us as parents to tune in to what's going on with our kids and their approach to food so that we can help them understand their own feelings, which may be creating or contributing to a disordered eating pattern. But we also need to understand our own emotions about food and eating so that we are able to get out of the way and give our children the structure and guidance that will fuel their confidence and faith in themselves.

The Picky Eater

The Picky Eater has a very limited palate. These children eat very few foods and may consume either very small amounts or a lot of what they do eat. They are completely unadventurous when it comes to trying new foods, and yet they can suddenly and with no apparent notice change their preference. They may, for example, eat nothing but chicken nuggets for months on end and then decide they "hate" them. What's important to understand about picky eaters is that most of the time, they really are getting all the nutrition they need (see the next chapter for specific nutritional guidelines).

Keep in mind that picky eaters are not being picky just to drive you nuts, but rather because they are very sensitive to the sensuality of foods—the taste, the texture, the smell, and the color or appearance of foods. Sometimes, the picky eater is also sensitive to things like the labels in his clothes. This same sensitivity to touch carries over into the realm of food. If you insist on picky eaters experimenting and trying to eat foods they won't tolerate, a struggle and fight will ensue. So before you go that route, stop and ask yourself, Why is this a problem? Is it a problem for me or my child? Recently, Margaret came to see me because her eight-year-old daughter, Sally, was very picky. In fact, according to Margaret, there was almost nothing Sally would eat. While the family had more or less figured out how to deal with this behavior, the girl's school was challenged by it, and her teachers were not sure what to do. In the back of her mind, Margaret confessed, she also had some worries about whether her daughter might be vulnerable to developing an eating disorder.

Sally was the youngest of three girls, and both her older sisters had been very adventurous eaters; in fact, Margaret told me, they were food enthusiasts who sometimes struggled with their weight. Sally, however, had always been tiny, short, and very, very thin. On the other hand, she was maintaining her growth curve, never got sick, and had energy to burn. Clearly, she was very healthy, and eating very few foods was not a problem for her, just the people around her (although her parents were managing quite impressively).

If Sally's parents had been less able to live with her picky eating and insisted on their daughter eating more varied foods, they could have created some serious power struggles. In general, I suggest giving picky eaters a bit more control, so that when their appetite drives their desire to experiment and try other foods, they will do so not to please you and not to rebel against you, but rather because their biology is telling them to. And keep in mind that Picky Eaters are annoying not because they are at risk but because it's hard for parents to watch them eat so few foods!

Tips for Dealing with Picky Eaters

- Reassure yourself that your child is getting adequate nutrition by making sure he (or she) is on the growth curve, has enough energy for all his activities, and is otherwise happy.

- Allow picky eaters to determine their own portion sizes. Even if they help themselves to only a little, try not to notice or comment. This way, children will feel less pressure to eat, tension will ease, and they will actually eat more.

- Continually model your own enthusiasm for different foods. Some families set a rule that everyone has to take one bite of a new food, but if they don't like it, they don't have to eat any more of it. This strategy seems to take the pressure off and offers children a way to get past their resistance to trying new things. If your child insists on not doing this, however, you may have to ask yourself, If she is healthy, is it worth the struggle? Very often picky eaters become less picky as they mature into young adulthood. Just keep reminding yourself that if your child is healthy, there really isn't a problem.

The Beige Food Eater

The Beige Food Eater is similar to the Picky Eater but eats only beige or white foods. They often start off eating everything, including vegetables, and then, when they turn two, seem to lose interest in any food with color. This preference for beige or white food can continue until children reach nine or beyond, but most Beige Food Eaters begin to expand their food horizons at about ten years of age.

Beige Food Eaters typically eat mainly carbohydrates, including breads, pasta, and cereal, although chicken nuggets and cheese are often favorites. Jane Guttenberg, M.D., says it is common for toddlers, who are just beginning to learn about their environment, to restrict their foods to those that seem bland or palatable. A young child is not making a conscious decision in this regard but rather, since food is yet another aspect of his expanding environment, he is trying to manage all these new stimuli. Here is a telling example. Elly, a mother of two children ages five and seven, stated that they had eaten all kinds of vegetables and fruits until they hit age two and a half; at that point, Elly tried every trick in the book—usually mashing up the carrots, broccoli, and so on, and hiding the vegetables in casseroles, in tomato sauce, or in whatever else she could think of—until, at age three, her daughter asked her, "Mommy, why is this mac and cheese green?" and Elly quickly realized that she was driving herself nuts.

The main concern for parents of this type of eater is whether or not their child is getting enough protein and/or fiber in his or her diet. But one pediatrician I consulted assured me that 99 percent of the time, the child is getting not only sufficient but plenty of nutrition. Again, if your child is healthy, on the growth chart, and doesn't seem to be lethargic (a sign of either low blood sugar or dehydration), you probably don't have much to worry about. Do, however, continue to offer your child access to all foods—even red, yellow, and green foods! Eventually she will become more comfortable with her entire environment and begin to explore new tastes.

Tips for Dealing with the Beige Food Eater

- Remind and reassure yourself that your child is getting adequate nutrition and that she will most likely grow out of this phase. It is very normal.

- Continue to model enthusiasm for varied foods, showing the Beige Food Eater that you, his siblings, and his friends love carrots and green beans. Show interest in the carrots the Beige Food Eater is not eating with statements such as, "Oh good, more for me!"

- You can also make smoothies that include yogurt, soy protein, or fruit in the beige color she likes! Pears, yellow apples, and white grapes are fruits that don't add too much color—who knows, she might like them!

The Spurt Eater

The parent of a Spurt Eater often finds himself or herself tense with anxiety: my child is going to starve to death! He never eats! The Spurt Eater is the kid who barely eats for days and then chows down like there's no tomorrow. Unfortunately, most parents of such eaters fail to either witness or keep track of how much food their child is actually eating. If you are such a parent, I want to assure you of two things: first, it's practically unheard of for a child to starve if he or she is given access to food on a regular basis; and second, your child is probably eating much more than you realize.

The first thing I advise parents of Spurt Eaters to do is to take an inventory. Literally, begin writing down the foods you see or know your child has eaten each day. Remember those four or five raisins? The six pieces of dry cereal? The granola bar on the way home from school? Such little snacks provide not only calories but also nutrition.

My three-year-old daughter, who is very thin, tends to be a Spurt Eater. (She is also quite picky but at times will branch out if she sees her sisters eating other things and asking for what she has left on her plate. You can always leverage the siblings!) At times I notice that she seems to have eaten very little for three days, and just as I'm beginning to ask myself if I need to worry or do anything differently, she always has a day when she requests a second bowl of cereal with milk. On those days, she even eats certain foods she usually won't touch, including turkey, salmon, and tons of fruit! Then she returns to her normal picky ways.

During her low-food phases, I continue to make all foods available to her and encourage her to try them, but I never push her too hard. I know she will eat when she is hungry, and my job is just to make sure the food is there when she wants it.

Tips for Dealing with the Spurt Eater

- When it appears as though your child is hardly eating, remember the days he plays catch-up and eats voraciously.
- Write down what your child eats for two weeks, or have your babysitter do this if it is too stressful for you.

Reminder!

- Remember that little bits add up for little bodies. Children do not need a lot of calories, and they do not need to eat complete or big meals in the same way adults do.
- Continue to model enthusiasm around eating. Again, adopt the attitude "Oh good, more for me!"
- Remember that everyone has hungry days and full days. Bodies are not machines and need both different amounts and different kinds of foods from day to day.
- Continue to establish mealtime not only as a time for eating but also as a time for enjoying one another's company, talking together, and laughing. Take the pressure away from eating if your children appear not to be hungry, but make sure to warn them that the kitchen is closing soon, so that you are not manipulated by the old "but I'm hungry" excuse right before, yes, you guessed it—BEDTIME!

The Grazer

The Grazer is yet another type of eater who drives parents crazy with worry about whether or not she is eating enough. The Grazer is the type of child who always nibbles but never sits down to a meal. Typically, Grazers are toddlers and preschoolers who seem to be happier eating tiny bits all day long rather than sitting down for three square meals a day. They are also children who tend to be easily distracted or to have shorter attention spans.

One of my clients, Lynn, was worried about her two-year-old daughter, Emma, who never sat down long enough to finish a meal. No matter how painstakingly Lynn prepared Emma's favorite foods—chicken nuggets with green beans, rice and beans, or pasta with red sauce—Emma would take a few bites and push her plate away. When I asked Lynn what Emma did next, she replied that her daughter usually just started playing with one of her toys. Sometimes she returned to her food; sometimes not.

I suggested that Lynn try a new strategy: instead of taking away Emma's plate of food once she had stopped or interrupted her own eating, Lynn would leave the plate someplace where Emma could easily see and access it. Soon after, Lynn called to report that, as I'd suspected, when she made the food available, Emma finished all the green beans, all the chicken nuggets, and all the rice—and she didn't seem to mind that her food was at room temperature!

Tips for Dealing with the Grazer

- If you're worried about your child's nutritional intake, write down what she actually eats for a two-week period (as with the Spurt Eater above).

- Allow mealtimes to extend a bit longer and do not expect her to sit for very long—especially if your child is a toddler.

- Be aware of the size of the snack bag you take to the park or on car trips. Are you contributing to your child's grazing habits? Do you think he cannot be without food for more than fifteen minutes? Are you being held hostage by his whines and your own fears that he might go hungry? If so, try to experiment with taking

Evaluating Whether Your Child May Have a Problem with Sensory Integration

WHILE SOME CHILDREN are just picky eaters, showing sensitivity to smells, textures, and the appearance of different foods, other children's sensitivity can be more extreme and part of a larger problem with sensory integration. These problems can show up in the Picky Eater, the Trouble Transitioner, the Beige Food Eater, and the Grazer. If you feel your child is showing signs of some of the following listed problems, I suggest you have him evaluated by an occupational therapist.

According to the Ayres Clinic, the founding research institution dedicated to problems in sensory integration, and Terry Sash, a speech pathologist and feeding therapist at Life Start, an early intervention program in New York City, the following are the signs of a sensory integration dysfunction:

- Overly sensitive to touch, movement, sights, or sounds. Does your child startle and appear unable to tolerate the usual loud sounds that others seem to be annoyed by, ignore, or manage?

- Underreactive to touch, movement, sights, or sounds.

- Easily distracted or showing extreme trouble with transitions.

- Social and/or emotional problems, including difficulty relating with peers and managing the intensity of the frustration that can come up when negotiating conflict, as displayed by unusually intense temper tantrums and aggression.

- Activity level that is unusually high or unusually low. Such a child can also appear to have low muscle tone and be less coordinated. He prefers to do most of his activities lying down and likes to lean on someone.

- Physical clumsiness or apparent carelessness, which can be a result of the slower development of the muscles and coordination that will impact on the oral/motor area of eating.

- Difficulty chewing, constant drooling, and breathing through an open mouth. He also has difficulty sipping through a straw by age two and takes a very long time to eat. Since managing food in the mouth is difficult, the child will begin to avoid eating foods that require chewing. He prefers liquids and softer foods.

- From eighteen to twenty-four months, she develops a severe pickiness about food, which can deteriorate into eating just two or three foods.

- The child chews food up and down rather than rotating food from one side of the mouth to the other, which is usually achieved by twenty-four months and is required for efficient chewing. Parents describe this difficulty chewing as "It seems he can only chew if I put food in just the right way and every couple of bites he just spits it out or gags."

- Extreme reactions to textures. He prefers only mushy or only crunchy, and the two textures cannot be mixed.

- Some history of gastric reflux and allergies. Some current experts think that a lot of sensory integration issues begin with gastrointestinal problems and also result from the body's rejection of foods to which it is highly allergic. Kids start to reject the texture of certain foods they might be allergic to because their bodies recognize that the food "doesn't feel safe."

- Impulsive, lacking in self-control.

- Inability to unwind or calm self.

- Poor self-concept.

- Delays in speech and language, and shows limited vocal sounds as a baby, uttering vowels and not incorporating consonants.

- Poor motor skills.

- Delays in academic achievement.

For a child to be classified as having a dysfunction in this area, he must exhibit a number of these qualities together, indicating a difficulty in several senses. The so-called normal Picky Eater will not exhibit all these signs together, but perhaps only two or three. You will know if your child has a more serious problem. I am a great believer in mother's intuition. Listen to the niggling worry in the back of your mind that, despite your doctor's reassurance that she is fine, you believe your daughter has a problem. My advice is to get a good evaluation with an occupational therapist to put your mind at rest. If your child is fine, then you can be reassured and move on. And if he does seem to have sensory integration problems, you can contact a private specialist or a free referral provided through a federal program that provides each state with funding. (See contact information in Resources.) Each state uses its money differently and functions independently. But again, early intervention can work wonders, helping to provide your child with added support in whatever area he needs it, whether it be speech development, occupational therapy, or both. These services will give him the necessary boost to continue on his path of development before he becomes self-conscious and aware of his difficulties in relation to other kids. Early intervention helps to avoid the development of low self-esteem in connection with these physiological difficulties.

fewer snacks and distract your child with other activities. You may see that he begins to eat more at one time, rather than spreading out through the day. Again, a child generally learns how to eat more at one time gradually as he moves through toddlerhood to preschool age.

- Even if your child doesn't eat much while sitting down for a meal, communicate that mealtime is not just for eating but also for enjoying one another's company. Continue to deemphasize your need for her to eat, but at the same time, don't let yourself be held hostage by the old "I'm hungry" routine just as bedtime arrives. I always say, "Come on, it's time for bed. You can always eat more tomorrow!"

What's Going On with Your Child?— A Review

As the last few chapters suggest, children's eating "problems" are usually not so much problems as they are side effects of their interaction with the world around them: their developmental stage, their temperament, and their eating style. What's important is to isolate the behavior itself and then consider some possible underlying factors. Here are some questions you can use as a guide:

- What age is your child?
- What is going on with the child developmentally?
- Which of the six eating styles is closest to your child's?

- Is this child different from his or her siblings?
- Is this child different from or similar to either you or your partner?
- Have you factored in your own food legacy?
- Are you worried about your child's becoming overweight?
- Is your child experiencing a growth spurt?
- Does your child have energy throughout the day?
- What does the pediatrician say about the child's weight in relation to his or her height? Is your child on the growth curve?

It's normal for parents to worry about whether their children are eating right, but as you go through these questions, keep in mind that a child's eating behavior or habit is always a function of at least two factors: their developmental stage and temperament traits. In the next chapter, you will take the first of four steps toward teaching kids how to eat for life. Step One will help guide you as you begin to talk to your child about nutrition. With this first step, he will begin the gradual process of learning about how different foods affect his body.

PART TWO

The Four Steps of Eating for Life

CHAPTER FOUR

Step One: Talk to Your Kids About Nutrition

It's important to remember that children have a remarkable inborn mechanism that lets them know how much food and which types of food they need for normal growth and development. It is extremely rare to see serious malnutrition or vitamin deficiency or infectious disease result from a feeding problem.

DR. BENJAMIN SPOCK,
DR. SPOCK'S BABY AND CHILD CARE

WE HAVE ALL PROBABLY arrived one time or another at the pediatrician's office with a mental list of questions: Is my child eating enough? Is she eating too much? How can I be sure my son is getting the proper nutrition? The pediatrician usually weighs and measures our child and then turns to us and says, "He's fine. He's on his growth chart. Relax." Relax? How can we possibly relax when it comes to our children's health?

All parents are concerned about how and what their children eat. After all, feeding our kids is usually the first and most concrete way we take care of our tiny vessels of life. And as they grow from babies to adolescents, our desire to feed them, strengthen them, and watch them grow healthy and wise only becomes stronger and more intense—while at the same time, their needs become more complicated. Indeed, they seem at times to thwart our every attempt to get them to eat "right."

We wouldn't be good parents if we didn't worry about our children's receiving proper nutrition. But in an era when we are inundated daily with nutritional information, our worry may be inflated out of all proportion to our actual need for concern. Some of this worry is the unintentional legacy of previous generations who experienced real, painful exposure to lack of nutrition. Indeed, many parents today were raised by either parents or grandparents who lived through the Great Depression of the 1930s or were immigrants from war-ravaged nations. These generations of Americans had good reason to be concerned about starvation and malnutrition. As pediatrician Dr. Jane Guttenberg says, "During the 1920s, 1930s, and 1940s, not getting enough food was a big deal; many kids really did die of malnutrition." And, consequently, it is "fed into our psyche that children are going to get sick if they do not get the proper nutrition."

Fortunately, in the United States today, food is abundant and malnutrition is rare. The majority of parents are able to provide their children with more than adequate food to meet their nutritional needs. Yet we have a host of other problems to contend with, among them a startling rise in obesity among children and adolescents.

So how do you as parents sort through all this nutritional information, help your children stay healthy, and put your minds at ease? Quite simply, you begin by talking to your kids about nutrition, teaching them about how different foods help their bodies to grow, their brains to stay sharp and focused, and their moods to stay as stable as possible. Children can and do learn how to take care of their bodies—but it requires a concerted effort on both their part and yours. If you are willing to make this effort, your children will begin to absorb the information, and slowly but surely they will integrate it so that they know a candy bar makes their tongue happy but it won't help their legs become stronger so they can run faster.

General Nutritional Guidelines for Kids

There is a lot of information available on how best to feed your kids. In 1999, the U.S. Department of Agriculture revised the Food Pyramid, and they also differentiated between the nutritional needs of adults and of young children. The Food Pyramid is a general guideline meant to show us how much of each type of food we should provide our children regularly. The *new* Food Pyramid for children recommends a varied diet that is high in green vegetables, grains, and legumes with moderate amounts of starchy carbohydrates and protein (meat, poultry, and fish), and small amounts of fat.

Take a look at the Food Pyramid for kids below, and use it as a general guideline for all children ages two to nine.

The Four Steps of Eating for Life

Food Guide Pyramid for Young Children

A Daily Guide for 2- to 6-Year-Olds

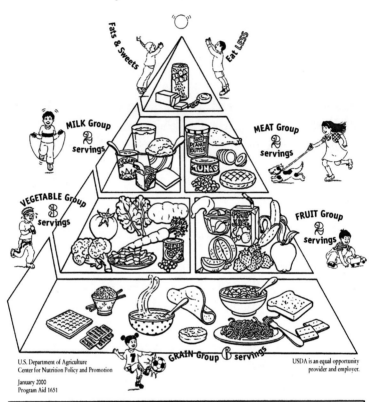

Fats & Sweets — Eat LESS

MILK Group
2 servings

MEAT Group
2 servings

VEGETABLE Group
3 servings

FRUIT Group
2 servings

GRAIN Group 6 servings

U.S. Department of Agriculture
Center for Nutrition Policy and Promotion

January 2000
Program Aid 1651

USDA is an equal opportunity
provider and employer.

WHAT COUNTS AS ONE SERVING?

GRAIN GROUP
1 slice of bread
½ cup of cooked rice or pasta
½ cup of cooked cereal
1 ounce of ready-to-eat cereal

VEGETABLE GROUP
½ cup of chopped raw or
cooked vegetables
1 cup of raw leafy vegetables

FRUIT GROUP
1 piece of fruit or melon wedge
¾ cup of juice
½ cup of canned fruit
¼ cup of dried fruit

MILK GROUP
1 cup of milk or yogurt
2 ounces of cheese

MEAT GROUP
2 to 3 ounces of cooked lean
meat, poultry, or fish

½ cup of cooked dry beans, or
1 egg counts as 1 ounce of lean
meat. 2 tablespoons of peanut
butter counts as 1 ounce of meat.

FATS AND SWEETS
Limit calories from these.

**Four- to 6-year-olds can eat these serving sizes. Offer 2- to 3-year-olds less, except for milk.
Two- to 6-year-old children need a total of 2 servings from the milk group each day.**

How to Use the Children's Food Pyramid

One of the easiest ways to begin to teach your children about nutrition and help them connect the foods they eat to their bodies' needs is to post a copy of the Food Pyramid on the refrigerator for easy reference. Or you can turn the lesson into an art project by having your children create their own Food Pyramid.

As you begin to talk about the different food groups and what they do for your child's body, refer to the Food Pyramid; the visual reference will help him make a more concrete connection between your words and the concepts themselves. And the shape of the pyramid itself will further reinforce the general recommendations for how much of each food group he should eat.

The Food Pyramid Is Not Static

I WOULD BE REMISS if I did not share with you that a number of nutritionists on the cutting edge of nutritional science are recommending that the bottom two rungs of the Food Pyramid be reversed: instead of recommending that most of a child's (or adult's) diet be made up of grains, they are recommending that children eat more vegetables and fruits. Also, many parents who are vegetarians and want to share this way of eating with their kids may wonder about safe guidelines. I suggest referring to the pioneering work of Charles R. Attwood, M.D., and his book *Dr. Attwood's Low-Fat Prescription for Kids,* as well as his website, www.vegsource.com.

Remember, however, that it's best to communicate the idea that no foods are bad; they just do different things for the body, and that's why it's best to eat more of some foods and less of others. This is especially true of the top rung, where sugar reigns supreme!

How Much Is Necessary?

While adequate portion sizes vary according to each child's body type, metabolism, and age, there are some consistent recommendations for how much children should eat of the three main food groups. Like adults, children should get at least 50 percent of their calories from carbohydrates, 30 percent from protein, and 20 percent (or less) from fats. And while many parents I speak to worry about regulating their children's portion sizes—some feel that their kids are eating too little and others worry that their kids are eating too much—it's crucial for you to keep in mind that what they eat is more important than how much. Without becoming too stressed, and with the understanding that no matter what your kids are eating their nutritional needs are probably being met, it's still a good idea to remember that quality is more important than quantity.

Unless your child has a pronounced eating disorder, or is very underweight or very overweight, you need to keep in mind that most kids get their nutritional needs met adequately on a biweekly basis. Again, kids do not have to eat three square meals each and every day to meet their nutritional demands.

Here are some basic guidelines suggested by the *Yale*

Guide to Children's Nutrition, as well as by renowned nutritionist Joy Bauer.

Protein

Protein is necessary for cellular growth and the proper synthesis of tissue such as muscle. Common kid-friendly sources of protein include eggs, milk, and dairy; meat, fish, and poultry; beans, soy products, and nuts. Here are some guidelines for what is considered an adequate protein supply:

Recommended Dietary Allowances for Childhood

CHILD'S AGE	BODY WEIGHT	GRAMS PROTEIN PER POUND	GRAMS PROTEIN PER DAY
0–6 months	13	1.00	13
7–12 months	20	.72	14
1–3 yrs	29	.54	16
4–6 yrs	44	.49	22
7–10 yrs	61	.45	28

Carbohydrates

Carbohydrates are a child's main source of energy, and without them children would not thrive or grow. Unfortunately, carbs are linked in many people's minds with foods that are "bad" or "fattening."

Carbohydrates are generally categorized as simple (sugars)—fruit juices, candy—and complex (multigrain breads and cereals, vegetables, and fruits). Complex carbohydrates are those that provide the best nutritional value and deliver

How Much Protein Is My Child Really Getting?

PARENTS NEED TO REALIZE how much protein their children are getting so they can relax.

- 8 ounces of breast milk contains 2.4 grams of protein.
- 8 ounces of commercial formula contains 4 grams of protein.
- 8-ounce sippy cup or glass of milk, including chocolate milk, contains 8 grams of protein.
- 1 ounce of cheddar cheese contains around 7 grams of protein.
- 1 tablespoon of peanut butter contains 4 grams of protein.
- 1 ounce of chicken, even in nugget form, contains 7 grams of protein.
- 8 ounces of yogurt contains 8 to 12 grams of protein.

the most usable energy. While there is no recommended dietary allowance (RDA) for carbohydrates, most experts recommend that 50 percent of children's calories be made up of mainly complex carbohydrates. Because kids have access to carbs in many different forms, nutritionists and pediatricians advise us that it's rarely necessary to worry about their getting adequate amounts.

Fat

Everybody—growing or not—needs an adequate supply of fat for cell membrane structure and important blood-clotting functions, as well as to deliver vitamins throughout the body. Fat cushions the organs and helps to circulate and absorb the fat-soluble vitamins A, D, E, and K. Fat is also what makes so many dishes we eat taste so good. There is, however, "good" fat and "bad" fat. The fat found in such foods as whole dairy, cream sauces, marbled meat, and baked goods that use butter, lard, cream, and hydrogenated vegetable oils are considered bad because they contain more saturated fat and trans-fatty acids, all of which contribute to high cholesterol and can lead to an increased risk for health concerns. Here are some general guidelines from the *Yale Guide to Children's Nutrition:*

AGE	GRAMS FAT	GRAMS SATURATED FAT
1–3 yrs	43	14 (or less)
4–6 yrs	60	20 (or less)
7–10 yrs	66	22 (or less)

Essential Vitamins and Minerals

We hear a lot about essential vitamins and minerals, but what exactly are they? For children, the most important include vitamins A, B, C, D, K, and iron and calcium.

Although some nutritionists and pediatricians advise parents to give their children a multivitamin, it is not because they really need it. In fact, many nutritionists with whom I spoke claimed that it was to create "peace of mind for the mommies." Most kids get what they need over a handful of days, so there is no need to worry. If you're very concerned that your children may not be getting enough essential vitamins because they have small appetites, don't eat

Make Dinner or Breakfast the Superstar Meal

NUTRITIONIST JOY BAUER recommends that parents try to make dinner their children's "superstar" meal. That way, they can see for themselves that their kids are eating healthfully and they'll be less inclined to worry all day about their nutritional needs. "Breakfast is second in line in importance," she says. "Between cereal and fortified waffles or eggs, kids are set." Again, breakfast and dinner are the meals we can control. If you can provide two out of three meals that are balanced, you can worry less about what is going on at or after school.

vegetables or fruit, or don't eat what you consider a well-balanced diet, by all means go ahead and give them a multivitamin to set your mind at ease. As nutritionist Jill Malden of New York City says, "It's far better for your child to have a relaxed mommy than a stressed-out mommy." But do remember the general rule of thumb: if your child is progressing appropriately on the growth chart in terms of height and weight, he is receiving adequate nutrition.

Talking to Your Kids About Foods

Use the following as general guidelines for how to start talking to your kids about different foods and how they help their bodies. The way you speak to your child depends a lot on how you communicate with that child on a daily basis, factoring in both her developmental stage and eating style, and your unique relationship with her. So while these suggestions have worked for many of my clients, you should feel free to adjust the wording, the tone, or the context to suit your particular situation. Keep in mind that it's best to tailor your examples to activities your child knows or enjoys. Your aim is to increase her motivation by helping her understand what the foods do for her, not for all other kids. So be specific and entice her interest by referring to individual interests and activities.

Ages Nine to Eighteen Months

While most children in this age group are not yet talking, you can still model your enthusiasm for eating a variety of foods and talk to them about how different kinds of foods work. Obviously, some of the conceptual information will be over their heads, but they will begin to hear the association between foods they eat and the impact those foods have on their bodies.

Keep in Mind

- While playing games with your baby, teach him the words for his body parts. For example, ask, "Where is Mommy's nose? Where is Johnny's mouth?" Point to the foods he is eating, saying, "Hmm, these carrots will help you climb the stairs" or "That milk you just drank is helping your body get taller so you can climb the steps to the slide in the playground all by yourself!"

- Make up your own version of the "head, shoulders, knees, and toes" game, and refer to foods as you do so.

- Begin to build in the idea that he knows when he is hungry and when he is full. If he stops eating and you're not sure he's had enough, see if he may have become distracted. You can offer him "one more bite," but try not to push it. You want your child to eat for himself, not for you. If he continues to refuse, say something like, "You must not be hungry. There is always more later." Make the food available and reoffer it an hour later. And remember, this age group can start to eat more sporadically, consuming a lot on one day and very little on another.

- Offer your child a range of foods and encourage him to feed himself. When he picks something such as cheese, for example, you can comment, "Yummy food! That will help you get taller!"

Sample Dialogue for Ages Nine to Eighteen Months

"Johnny! You climbed all the way to the top of the slide this morning! I saw you! Did you realize that this piece of cheese made your legs longer so you reached that rung? And this piece of chicken made your muscles bigger in your arms and legs, so that you were able to get all the way to the top and had all that energy to play for so long this morning! Show me where your arm bone is. Do you want some more milk so you can help your bones grow? Boy, you are helping your body do fun things!"

"Annie, you got in and out of the sandbox all by yourself this afternoon! You are so much bigger now that you can climb and walk! You have helped yourself grow taller with this yogurt you love and the milk you had this morning! And this apple you're eating now is keeping you strong so that you can play in the playground tomorrow, too!"

"Joey, you have so much energy to walk and run! I could barely keep up with you! This cracker and this orange are going to keep giving you energy to play even more. And look at this muscle; show me your muscle! Wow! Your muscles are growing because of the turkey you had at lunch and all these great foods; you are such a great captain of your body!"

Ages Eighteen Months to Three Years

At the beginning of this stage, from ages one and a half to two years old, children are often less adventurous with food. They tend to eat when hungry and not eat when they're not. Parents often describe their children never eating a "full meal" but rather "grazing" throughout the day. However, children in this age group are more verbal and can start to comprehend and talk more specifically about how foods impact their bodies.

Keep in Mind

- Keep talking in terms they can relate to about how various foods help their bodies grow. Talk about their bodies being like engines, and how foods with protein fill up their engine so that it runs smoothly and they can play longer. Explain how all the foods with vitamins and carbs also give the engine fuel. Kids love the fuel and car or train analogy. If they are demanding sugar, teach them how sugar is like giving their engines a teeny bit of gas, and explain how other, more nutrient-rich foods will give them a fuller tank.

- You know your child; focus on the activities she loves to do physically. For example, point to the carrots that help give her energy to run.

- You can begin to use words such as *protein* and *calcium,* but don't worry too much about this terminology. It's more important at this stage to begin to move away from the vagueness of "this will help your body grow" and speak more specifically about how particular foods function in helping their bodies do the activities they love.

- Reinforce the idea that they are taking good care of their bodies by eating so well. Begin to teach them that they are not only the EXPERTS on their bodies but that it is also their JOB to take good care of their bodies.

Sample Dialogue for Ages Eighteen Months to Three Years

"Karl, let's look at this beautiful drawing of the Food Pyramid Mom made for the refrigerator door so we can figure out what you might want to have for lunch: what is in the fridge that matches the drawing?"

"Casey, do you want to have a playdate with Anna? Do you want to play with that new game Grandma bought you? Great! Did you know that this peanut butter sandwich is going to help you play for as long as you want? It's what helps your brain think and keeps your tummy full so you won't have to stop."

"Are you hungry again? Boy, you must be growing

right now! Let's look at the foods on our Pyramid and figure out what might help your tummy stay full and also help those bones and muscles keep growing! Help me pick what you want to eat."

"I see that your feet just grew into those princess shoes you love! Look at what a great job you are doing! You drank your milk and cheese, and even that broccoli helped your feet grow to fit into those shoes!"

Ages Three to Five Years

This stage is very much characterized by children's wanting to establish even more separateness, independence, and power—a struggle that is played out with (or against) their parents. Understandably, kids in this age range continue to assert their will with relation to food, and that willfulness often results in struggles between children and parents around establishing and following guidelines, especially concerning sugar. This is a great age to make the Food Pyramid into an art project. If your children are not inclined to draw, suggest that they cut out different foods from magazines and paste them into the big triangle they drew themselves. As you do this, you can teach them about what the foods do, and also why it is good to fill up their stomach with more of some of these foods than others.

Keep in Mind

- You can now begin to use words like *protein, vitamins,* and *calcium* and to explain what they do for your child's body. Explain how cheese, for example, is a good source of calcium, and fish is a good source of protein. Make sure to follow up by telling them how these foods make their bones grow so they can fit into that princess dress they love so much, or how they will help their legs grow to climb that slide in the park.

- Defuse power struggles and continue to build children's motivation to take care of their own bodies by letting them make some food choices on their own.

- Try to avoid the old "eat one more bite and then you can have dessert." This is difficult and at times hard not to fall into—especially if you have been getting your child to eat his veggies by stalling on the dessert. But remember that your goal is getting your children to begin taking responsibility for their bodies. Again, reinforce the idea of filling up on foods that will do good things for their bodies: "Hmm, I know you don't want the broccoli, and you can't wait for dessert, but what do you think you need to eat to do good things for your body? Dessert is fun and tastes terrific, but what can you also eat that will help you run around during playtime at school tomorrow?" Remind your children that they are the experts on their bodies and they are the only ones who know from the inside when they are hungry and when they are full.

- Begin to build in ways for your kids to think about how they have eaten and taken good care of themselves each day. Kids are used to either eating or not eating the foods we put in front of them and just following what we tell them to do. By helping them to think about how they have fed themselves, you begin to instill the idea that it is their job to think about the foods they have had over the course of the day. This way you start to develop their sense of responsibility toward their own bodies, particularly at a time when they are proud of their growing independence and autonomy. Once they grasp that concept they will feel motivated to make some decisions about how to eat.

- Encourage them to tell you which foods help strengthen their bodies. Check that they really understand what particular foods do for them: Reinforce the concepts of protein for muscle growth and concentration, vitamins for all-over growth, calcium for bone growth, and carbs for energy. Point out that sugar is also great, but it won't help their bodies grow and stay strong.

Sample Dialogue for Ages Three to Five Years

"I know you want more cookies, and I agree they taste really good! They make your tongue happy, so it makes sense that you want more of them. But let's figure this out. If you fill your stomach with nothing but cookies, how are you going to play this afternoon? Your tongue will be happy now, but your body won't have any fuel! Let's see if we can pick something to eat that you know will fuel your body. Help me out here. Then, if you still want it, you can always have a cookie later."

"I know we had to end that playdate because Johnny got tired and cranky. He was hungry. Are you? Do you know that these carrots you just had and that mac and cheese will help you play as long as you want? Good job! You are doing so well taking care of your body!"

"I know you're sad that those Rollerblades Uncle Dave got you don't fit yet. But let's keep those bones growing.

Those strawberries and the milk you had with your cereal will help you grow to fit into those Rollerblades. It will happen; you are going to keep those bones growing strong because you are so smart! Let's look at this drawing Mom made that we put up on the fridge. What other foods help your bones grow?"

Ages Five to Seven Years

This age group tends to eat more, sometimes all day long. At times parents may also notice dramatic shifts in tastes. One week your child loves peanut butter and the next, he hates it. Depending on the child's size and rate of growth, parents should also expect variations in appetite. And keep in mind that children will continue to test limits around guidelines, particularly once they enter school, begin having playdates, and are, therefore, more exposed to different families and styles.

Keep in Mind

- You can continue to reinforce what you've been teaching your children about various foods in a more sophisticated way. For example, you can explain that protein helps sustain their concentration so they can do their work in school; that calcium is important for growing taller; and that carbs are essential for energy and concentration—both in school and during recess. You can also emphasize the fact that they need calcium for healthy teeth. They are losing their baby teeth and getting adult teeth at about this age, and it's a big deal to them, so do capitalize on that.

- Continue to increase your child's motivation to take good care of her body, and emphasize her growing maturity by letting her make some food choices.

- Reinforce her growing ability to integrate the nutritional information you are teaching her by commenting on how well she is caring for herself and how responsible she is being. Continue to respect her choices if you see that she is eating well overall and occasionally wants a dessert or sweet treat. Try not to be too rigid, so that you teach her how to be flexible.

- Some children even at this age, but more so in the next stage, are beginning to worry that they are fat. Help them include the foods they love and not be too hard on themselves. Children who are very rigid and tend to be perfectionists might begin to become self-critical of their bodies and how they eat. Try to help them be moderate, and explain why it is important for them to be satisfied so that they do not overeat.

Sample Dialogue for Ages Five to Seven Years

"Rory, I know you want more dessert. How do you think that tooth is doing that's coming in now? Are you being nice to that tooth? Do you think you might have had too much sugar? Are you helping that tooth grow well by eating enough calcium? Here are the things you can eat that have calcium; you take your pick."

"Johnny, I know you never want to eat breakfast. You are never hungry when you wake up, but you are always starved while we're walking to school! So let's pick two things you can eat while we go to school that will give you energy all day. That turkey you had in your sandwich yesterday has protein that will give you concentration and keep you full. Yes, the bagel will give you energy, too, but if you add turkey, it can help you stay full longer. Let's put it in a bag to eat on the way."

"Would you like to eat that waffle hot or cold? I can heat it up for you if you want, and then we'll put it in this bag to eat along the way."

"I know you hate vegetables, and that's too bad because vegetables have so many of the vitamins your body really needs to help it stay strong and do things like skating. But fruit is also really great, and it has a lot of vitamins, too, so let's pick some fruits you love, and then maybe when you want to try some vegetables we can find one you don't hate."

Ages Seven to Nine Years

Since children are developing more intellectual maturity at this age, they are better able to integrate nutritional information and to enjoy taking responsibility for their own bodies. This is, therefore, a great stage for parents to give kids greater responsibility for making their own food choices and to allow for more flexibility in their responses to such questions as, "Mom, can I have this cookie?"

Keep in Mind

- Continue to dialogue with your kids about nutrition and enjoying their food. Turn their questions into ones they can answer for themselves. For example, when they ask, "Mom, can I have this?" ask in response, "What do you think? Shall we think about it together to see what your body might be needing?" (Of course, you will not do this all the time, but even if you do it sometimes, you are reinforcing your children's thought processes and decision-making skills, and you are increasing their motivation to use the information they have about nutrition.) Offer your support but don't make the decision for them. Sometimes they will want your help, sometimes not. By allowing them to make their own decisions and observing how they do that, their confidence will build, as will yours.

■ Remember that teaching kids how to eat for life is a process, and not all days will be perfect. Sometimes your child will be tired and just want you to tell him what to do. Some days, you will want to tell him what to eat, or say "no" because it won't make sense to have a dialogue at that moment. Sometimes you will have to be more involved and remind your child of the limits. You may also have to point out that if he has three bowls of ice cream, he is not acting very responsibly toward his body. Again, continue to reinforce his understanding that you expect him to want to take care of himself because it is his body. And you can help him, but it is really his job to take good care of it.

Sample Dialogue for Ages Seven to Nine Years

"Dana, would you help me do some grocery shopping this week? You have become such an expert on these foods and what your body needs. I also really want you to help me pick what you like, because your tastes keep changing; I thought you loved salmon! So I need you to help me pick another food you might like that contains good protein. I know you loved finishing that book you wanted to read! We want to keep that brain going strong and give you good concentration! Protein really helps with that."

"Sarah, I know you take great care of your body by giving it a lot of vitamins and protein, and carbs for energy. But you won't tell me what foods you'd like to give you calcium for your bones and teeth. What's going to happen? You'll have great strong muscles but bad bones and teeth? Help me out here. I know you hate milk, cheese, and yogurt, but we have got to figure something out."

"I know you love that Frappuccino, and it does taste great. But it's like having three candy bars for dessert. Do you want your Frappuccino now or would you rather wait until after dinner when you have had some other food to fill up on?"

"I understand that you want to be a vegetarian, but you still have to make sure your body gets enough protein, so you will have to help me figure out which foods you like and how much you will need of them. Do you still want to eat fish? Chicken? What meat exactly are you saying you want to stop eating? Okay, let's find some other protein options to keep your brain and muscles going."

The Perils of Making Sugar into a Treat or Taboo

Help! is what most parents say in desperation when it comes to the sugar cry from their children. "What should I do when my kids constantly ask for candy? I know it's not good for them to eat too much sugar, but that's all they want!" Once your children are exposed to the world at large—through playgroups, at school, at friends' homes, and so on—you are no longer in total control of their foods. Typically, this increased exposure happens after about three years old, when kids enter preschool. But it can happen earlier for your second child. Even if you were able to keep your first baby away from sugar, your second is usually exposed much earlier on because of his older sibling's exposure to sugar. For many parents, trying to find a way to help manage their children's intake of candy, cookies, and desserts becomes a very frustrating challenge. But there are ways to deal with the sugar dilemma, no matter how uncomfortable you may be with kids' general desire for sweets.

Again, it's important that no food be declared bad or good. Rather, those that are less nutritious, such as sugary foods, can be described as "fun for the tongue" or as "food that makes your taste buds happy." When children learn that a food is forbidden, they quite naturally become more curious about and drawn to that food, sometimes even becoming obsessive about it. This is the case with the six-year-old child who will eat only Fluffernutter sandwiches for lunch, the five-year-old who can't stop eating from the box of Krispy Kreme donuts, or the four-year-old who can eat bowl after bowl of ice cream with sprinkles!

Of course, eating sweets in moderation is key. If, in general, your children eat nutritious food, a couple of days of eating doughnuts and candy is not going to kill them. But that doesn't help us stay calm, cool, and collected when our children seem to want to eat nothing but candy or junk food! Children who overeat sugary foods can drive parents crazy with worry.

It is my belief that most children can learn to eat all foods in moderation if they are given proper guidelines about nutrition and enough access to all varieties of food, including sugar. I also realize, however, that while some kids will be happy with a couple of pieces of candy or one or two cookies, others have more difficulty finding their sugar stopping point. There is no doubt that some children, like some adults, have more of a sweet tooth than others. But even those children who seem unable to stop their craving can be taught how to eat sweet foods in moderation. These desired foods, however, cannot be made forbidden or taboo.

While I know how difficult it is to stay away from the old "Take one more bite of broccoli and then you can have dessert" routine, avoiding the use of treats as rewards for any kind of accomplishment, good behavior, or finishing all the food on the plate is important if you don't want to make sugar more desirable than other foods in the minds of your children. If, for example, you reward your child with dessert for finishing dinner or eating his vegetables, you are only reinforcing the negative associations he might have with dinner and vegetables and creating positive, taboo associations around dessert. If, instead, children are taught that sweet foods have their own characteristics just like any other foods, then they will be less likely to think of such foods as special. The point is to not make sugar more desirable than other foods. Remember, all foods are good!

It's also dangerous to insist that your child have "just a taste" of his vegetables in order to have dessert, especially if he seems to be developing an aversion to vegetables or any other food. In fact this approach will simply lessen the chance that he will ever grow to like the food you are trying to get him to eat. Most children will be so focused on

Avoid Making Food a Reward

ACCORDING TO RECENT STUDIES by child development experts, parents who use food as a reward or make a favorite activity contingent upon eating certain foods (vegetables, for example) may be "making short-term gains with long-term losses." Here are the results of one particular study in which preschoolers were given certain snacks, including juice, over a four-week period and rewarded for eating previously rated neutral snacks. Children were rewarded either by verbal praise ("That's very good, you drank your juice all the way down") or by a ticket to a ten-minute children's movie ("Okay, you drank it, you get a ticket to the movie") for drinking a juice the child had rated neutral in a prior taste preference test. Researchers found that the children liked the juice less rather than more as a result of being rewarded for eating it. "The findings are consistent with what has been called the over-justification hypothesis (Lepper & Greene, 1978), which suggests that sometimes the persistent use of a contingent reward may overjustify an activity. In this case, praise overjustifies drinking the juice, which leads the child to discount its value. As one child put it, 'When Mom tells me I can't have my dessert until I clean my plate, what's left on my plate is usually yucky' (Birch, Marlin, & Rotter, 1984, p. 438). Rewards often have a paradoxical effect and may decrease rather than increase preferences!" (From *Child Psychology, A Contemporary Viewpoint,* E. Mavis Hetherington, Ross D. Parke, 3rd Edition.)

the sweet they really want that they will never realize they actually like the taste of the baked potato or carrots and snap peas that are being presented as an obstacle to the dessert. It's up to you as parents to reinforce—constantly and consistently—the idea that our bodies need all foods and that it's the child's job to take care of her own body. I encouraged one parent to try this with her four-year-old who had a real sweet tooth and always resisted eating any of the vegetables the family was having for dinner. So one evening, instead of falling for her daughter's query of "How many more bites do I need to take before dessert?" the mother simply reminded her daughter that she should know. "You are a big girl now," she said. "You are learning how to take care of your body. What do you think?" Because she shifted the responsibility to her daughter and resisted the urge to answer the question herself, the daughter ended up taking four more bites—certainly more than she would have eaten if her mother had stayed involved in the decision.

If sugar has been made neither a taboo nor a treat, children learn to relax around it and will be less likely to turn to such foods in an obsessive way. Maybe one child does gravitate more toward sugar and demands it more often than another; maybe one doesn't get as full as quickly as another. But most children will eventually become bored with the cake or cookies if they are allowed access to them. To appreciate the truth of this, you need only observe the child who never gets to have candy devour her bag of treats on Halloween while children who are always allowed access to candy tend to eat some and save the rest for later.

Setting Sweet Parameters

Children do need parameters, and very few parents are comfortable with giving their children complete access to candy and sweets at all times. If you are someone who is more concerned about regulating or limiting sugar intake, it's very important that you honor and respect those feelings and beliefs. This is true for some of the parents with whom I work, who for health, medical, or moral reasons feel more comfortable being more restrictive around sugar. Depending on where you feel comfortable on the sugar continuum, here are some suggestions about how to deal with your kids and sugar:

1. If sugar intake is a health issue, educate your children, making sure they understand that they are harming their health by eating anything sweet. Help them find other foods that feel to them like treats.
2. Let them have a sweet once or twice a week, but they get to pick the day.
3. If one treat per day is acceptable to you, let your children choose the time, as long as they eat other foods that fuel the body. Even if they choose to eat their sweet at breakfast, remind them that this is their choice and they are saying they want it now instead of later on in the day, or after dinner, with the rest of the family.
4. Allowing treats more than once a day is also an option. The decision is all about the balance between overeating and undereating. Stay aware of how your child manages his treats. Is he overeating or undereating other, more nutritious foods? If not, then he does not have a prob-

lem with sugar and more than likely will not be requesting three treats every day!

5. You can impose your beliefs about sugar for only so long. You therefore need to realize that your child will soon be able to start sneaking it at other people's homes or eating it outside your home if you are too rigid. In order to avoid this secretive eating, see if you can build in a bit more flexibility so that you are helping him make decisions about sugar while he is still at an age when he will absorb that information from you. Then, when he is able to access all the sugar he wants, he will be familiar and comfortable with the idea of moderation.

6. Explain that sometimes our body tricks us into thinking all we want is sugar when in fact it needs something else. Why? Because when we feed our body sugar or starches (both simple and complex carbohydrates), we can trigger a craving for more and more. If you respond this way to carbs, your child may have inherited the same sensitivity, making the craving for sugar intense. Reinforce the importance of feeding his body foods that will help it to grow. Let him know you understand that sugar is also important for fun, but that he needs to feed his hunger with other foods. Once he does that, he can always have the sweet, too.

The waiting game is also useful to help teach kids that their tongues might be telling them they want another cookie when what they really need is a break. See what happens when they learn to wait ten to fifteen minutes so that their body has a chance to let their brain know whether or not they really want more. (You will find more advice on this in Step Two.)

7. Try suggesting that the sugar they want may really be a way to satisfy another desire, such as attention from you or your spouse, wanting to do something else, or an expression of being bored, tired, or frustrated. If children learn to connect to their feelings, they will be less likely to think they are hungry when they're really not. (You will find more advice on this in Step Three.)

When Kids Can't Seem to Stop

We know that, by and large, babies do self-regulate (you will learn more about this phenomenon in chapter five). However, many parents worry that their children will not continue to self-regulate as they get older, especially when sugar enters the picture. In fact, some children do show much more interest than others in sweet foods and will tend to eat more without stopping. If you think your child may be having difficulty self-regulating around sugar, consider the following tips:

1. Examine your rules with regard to sugar. Are they too restrictive or rigid? Have you provided any access to sweet foods?
2. Give your child more control over when and what sweets he can choose, but define your guidelines and state them clearly to your child.
3. Review the nutritional characteristics of the various foods on the Food Pyramid.
4. Encourage him to take an interest in caring for his own body.

5. Try the Waiting Game exercise (page 132) to reinforce your child's ability to pay attention to the signal between his stomach and his brain. Then ask him if his stomach still wants more of the sweet food.

6. Try distracting your child with an activity you know he likes, reassuring him that the treat or dessert will always be there for him at another time.

7. Help him figure out the difference between wanting the additional ice cream and what he might really be feeling. Is he hungry for the ice cream or does he really need a hug? Is he upset about something else in his life?

A Last Resort

If you are dealing with a child who is relentless in his demand for sugar, and all your attempts to help him eat moderately have failed, you can try this next step. I am warning you, however, that it is not for the faint of heart, and the only people I have worked with who are willing to try it are those at the end of their rope. Still, if you're able to follow through, it will be the ultimate cure. There is one caveat: if your child has an underlying medical problem or condition, such as diabetes or food allergies, this approach is contraindicated, and you need to consult with your medical practitioner and a nutritionist to help establish safe and realistic guidelines.

Begin with the seven steps above, and then continue:

8. Let him pick a dessert he is always demanding—let's say, Oreo cookies. Tell him he can have as much or as many as he wants; there is no limit. He can eat the

Oreo cookies day and night if he would like, even to the exclusion of all other foods. (I told you, you have to have guts to do this!) In fact, tell him that he should make sure he always has Oreo cookies on hand so he won't run out. The key idea here is that your child should not be Oreo-deprived.

9. Observe what happens. You need to be prepared for the eventuality that your child might eat Oreos nonstop for several days or even a week. Try not to notice how much he is eating or you will be worried, and he may observe that you are not trusting the process. Even if he eats an entire box of cookies, it is more than likely that by the second week he will be eating fewer cookies, and fewer still after that.

10. If you try this approach, it is highly unlikely that your child won't at a certain time lose interest in the Oreo cookies. I have used this strategy to cure hundreds of individuals of their belief that certain foods have power over their bodies. If you do try it, however, you need to know that, in the short run, your child may gain weight. (For more information on this subject, see *Overcoming Overeating*, by Jane R. Hirschmann and Carol H. Munter).

11. However, if after three weeks there appears to be no end in sight, and your child is eating only boxes and boxes of Oreo cookies, he is clearly incapable of self-regulating, and you need to admit to yourself and to him that this is not working. Although it happens rarely, a child who has no connection to his body's signals will have to be provided with a structured way of eating that is completely imposed from without. Dis-

cuss this openly and in a matter-of-fact way, helping your child to understand that the Oreo experiment was a fact-finding mission to help him learn more about his body, its needs, and its appetites. Point out that his body does not appear to give him a signal of satiety for sweets, and that he is going to have to follow guidelines to take good care of his body for life. If he is unable to follow these guidelines, and you are looking for additional help because you are worried about how to help him learn to stop, consult with a nutritionist and/or a therapist who specializes in eating issues.

12. Understand that to your child these guidelines will, of course, feel like restrictions. Educate him and try to get him on board with the idea that both of you have the same goal, which is to help him to do the things he loves to do, including keeping his body running and growing as efficiently as possible.

A Quick Review

As you begin talking to your kids about nutrition, keep in mind it's a gradual process that takes time and patience—on both your part and your children's. Kids learn and retain information a little bit at a time—and sometimes seem to forget everything all at once! Don't despair. This strategy does work and will work for you. Just remember:

- Eating well does not mean eating well every single day. Children's nutritional needs are met on a one- to two-week basis and not day to day or meal to meal. Not every meal has to include all of the food groups, especially if your kids are small and have small appetites!

- Use realistic standards, and incorporate flexibility. These are the building blocks that will help your child to maintain healthy eating habits for life.

- Kids learn to integrate the information you are teaching them in a gradual way; don't expect them to suddenly wake up after just a week or two and know how to eat for life.

- Model the eating behavior you would like your children to emulate, and remember to monitor your own negative comments about food or eating. Children will model this behavior, as well as the attitude behind it.

- No matter how clear you are, no matter how flexible or strict you are, there will be days when your children are simply offtrack when it comes to eating and food.

I am a big believer in balance and moderation. There is a trend in this country at the moment toward eating more protein and fewer carbohydrates. I, however, feel strongly that the rigid restriction of any food does not result in good health over the long run and, furthermore, results in too much obsessing about what to eat and what not to eat. In a nutshell, restriction promotes disordered eating and does not help free one from thinking about food. I have seen this over and over not only in my practice but also in my conversations with men and women who spend a lot of time thinking about their food intake that could be better used to enjoy their food, among other pursuits.

If we treat our children as if they don't know how to

take care of themselves, they will not learn. They will rely on us to do so, or they will rebel against us. Creating this dialogue will help build their self-esteem as they sense your pride in their competence at making good and sound nutritional decisions. And, again, it's key not to be rigid! Sound nutrition is achieved through good general habits. If good habits are in place, the body can tolerate variations. This is what we want our children to learn by taking ownership of nutrition—good habits that will sustain them for a lifetime of eating.

CHAPTER FIVE

Step Two: Reboot the Connection Between the Belly and the Head

Weight and height must be considered together to determine whether a child is overweight. If that child is also at the ninety-fifth percentile for height, then the weight is fine.

THE YALE GUIDE TO CHILDREN'S NUTRITION

My mother was always saying to me: "Haven't you had enough?" It always bothered me, and I don't want to do that to my daughter, but I worry when I see her taking second and third helpings! Especially with all this concern about children and obesity; how do I trust that she knows when she's had enough?

MOTHER OF AN EIGHT-YEAR-OLD

ALL CHILDREN COME INTO this world with an innate sense of what their bodies need. They know when they're hungry; they know when they're full. They know when to start eating and when to stop because they are hardwired to receive a built-in signal that delivers messages from the body to the head. As children leave babyhood, however, this signal can become

119

harder to hear, and the communication between the belly and the brain can break down. If a child's body is telling him he doesn't want to eat anymore, but his mother is encouraging him to have one more bite because she's fearful that he hasn't had enough, how is the child to continue to interpret his own signal of fullness? Should the child begin to believe that his mommy hears the signals from his tummy better than he? The problem here is this: if what Mommy thinks he should eat is more than his body needs, the child might begin to associate fullness with a feeling of being stuffed, which in turn can lead to overeating.

It is for this reason that parents need to pay attention to their children's cues and not be guided only by their own worries about whether or not their children are eating too little or too much. It is our job as parents to help our kids stay connected to their bodies' signals, or, if those signals have gone awry, to help reboot the connection between their bellies and their brains.

In this chapter, you will learn how to reboot that connection by teaching your children to tune into their degree of hunger and fullness using the Hunger-Fullness scale, and to understand what it feels like to be sated—satiety is the key to eating moderately, neither too little nor too much. Once they learn to recognize these feelings, children will also come to understand that they (not their parents) are the experts on their own bodies and that it's up to them to take care of their bodies. Let's take a look at the importance of this connection between the belly and the head.

Communication Breakdown

Babies are born with the ability to self-regulate, and we as parents hear their signals loudly and clearly: they scream to be fed, and we feed them. Indeed, during the first three months of a baby's life we have full license to demand feed our infants. And many parents derive a great sense of satisfaction from being able to tune in and respond to their babies' signals so easily.

Further down the road, however, when the baby begins to eat solid foods more regularly and parents are encouraged by their pediatricians to wean him from the bottle, they begin to doubt their child's ability to eat when hungry and stop when full. No longer able to rely on the nutrition they know is provided by formula or breast milk, they worry, How will I know if she is getting enough? How will I know he is getting his nutritional needs met? And especially, If he doesn't eat enough food, then his sleep may be interrupted, and he will wake up hungry in the middle of the night! Ironically, it is this very worry that may lead parents to interfere with or override their own kids' signals, unwittingly causing them to become confused about what their own bodies are telling them.

One couple consulted with me because the father was worried that his wife was not feeding their fourteen-month-old enough food. I remember his announcing proudly, "John always eats more with me!" His concerns were twofold: that their son began waking up because he didn't eat a lot and therefore wasn't eating enough, and that he might become hungry in the middle of the night. The wife, however, felt very tuned in to her son's signals and didn't think that the few occasions when he did awaken during the night were attributable to hunger. She also hated the thought of "trying to get him to eat more" because she remembered being pushed to eat by her own mother and grandmother as a youngster and hating it. Their difference of opinion on this issue began to cause contention between them, and the longer it continued, the more the mother began to mistrust her own instincts about whether her son was really full when he stopped eating.

While it certainly would not be the end of the world if the boy ate a bit more, I wanted the couple to make sure they were respecting their son's connection between his belly and his head. Most of the time, babies stop eating when they are full. If we try to feed them more than their belly is saying to take in, children learn the following: (1) When I eat, it makes Mommy and Daddy happy, so I should eat for them, (2) Mommy and Daddy must know my body better than I do, so I should disregard this signal from my belly telling me I am full.

These mixed signals undermine the child's ability to self-regulate and lead him to pay less attention to the signals from his belly to his head. Despite the loud and clear signal saying, "I AM FULL NOW. I DON'T NEED TO EAT ANYMORE," the child will begin to disregard the messages from his belly. The signal will then become muted, leaving the child in the difficult position of not knowing when he's supposed to stop eating—when he has finished his portion? when Mommy looks happy?—or when he feels full?

Another problem this situation sets up is that the child learns to eat with his eyes or head, as opposed to eating from his stomach. I call this external versus internal eating. External eating means paying more attention to outside factors when determining when and what to eat. Internal eating means eating according to the needs of one's individual body. I always coach parents and tell children: "The information is all there. It is all in your body. You are the expert, but at times you may have to be a really good detective to figure out what your body is telling you. Sometimes the signals are loud, and sometimes they are soft. But let's see if you can close your eyes and listen carefully to what your body might be saying."

All that said, however, I don't want you to worry that anytime you urge your children to eat a bit more to make sure they have had enough, you are setting up a problem. In fact, it was unlikely that the parents I just described were going to create a serious problem for their son. In the end, the father did listen when his son shook his head and displayed an utter lack of interest in eating any more. The more important concern was that the mother had lost confidence in her ability to tune in to her son, which could, in the long run, do more damage than trying to overfeed him.

Indeed, as soon as a child is about a year old and eating solids, there is a push from pediatricians and other parents toward getting him to eat three meals a day with snacks in between. The idea is to help the child participate in mealtimes so that he is part of the social fabric of the family and the larger world. It is during these years when many children lose their ability to self-regulate. They eat to make their parents happy; they eat because they are temperamentally easygoing and compliant and know that this is what you want from them. Or, conversely, they are very strong-willed, and

Does Hunger Interrupt Sleeping Through the Night?

AS PARENTS BEGIN to wean children from the breast or the bottle, they often worry that the child may wake up hungry, particularly if she doesn't eat a lot. If that worry then motivates the parent to feed her child during the night, she may well begin to undo whatever sleep training she's managed to set in motion. As pediatrician Jane Guttenberg, M.D., of New York City states, "If children eat in the middle of the night, they will just develop that habit, become used to eating then, and continue to expect it. This is similar to when you are on vacation and your body gets used to having breakfast at 11 A.M. It quickly becomes a habit. But parents can break that habit, and children do not need to eat in the middle of the night."

it's easy for them to use eating as a way to gain control and define themselves as different from you. Whatever a particular child's eating behavior, it's critical that you as the parent pay attention to whether your child is still connected to his signals of hunger and fullness. You know your children and you are in the best position to help them maintain confidence in their ability to read their own signals.

The Hunger-Fullness Scale for Children

When kids are having trouble determining their degree of hunger or fullness, I've found it helpful to use a Hunger-

Fullness scale I've adapted from Debra Waterhouse's very useful and insightful book for women, *Outsmarting the Female Fat Cell,* as a way to teach them how to assess their hunger and/or fullness. I encourage parents to sit with their children, discuss what the numbers on the scale mean, and then let the kids describe their own interpretation of the scale, using colors and their own words.

The Scale

7. "I'm stuffed." (extremely full to the point of discomfort or pain)
6. "I'm full." (full to the point of feeling bloated)
5. "I'm done." (comfortably sated)
4. "I'm not sure if I'm hungry." (Need to wait a bit longer to get a louder reading of the signal)
3. "I'm hungry." (first signal that your body needs food)
2. "I'm starving." (strong signal to eat, very hungry)
1. "I feel sick." (irritable or dizzy, often past the point of reading the signal as hunger)

One of the most important uses of this scale is to teach your children the lesson that in order to feed their bodies well and not under- or overeat, they need to keep tuning in to the numbers 3 and 5. Number 3 is a healthy signal of hunger. You want to help kids learn not to wait to eat until they are starving (number 2), although this sometimes will happen. We all know the signs that small children are at number 1: they begin to melt down right before our eyes. And because it is more difficult to get this group to sit down to eat, it's particularly important to help them read their signals so that they will eat before they reach this point.

Then if they learn to stop eating when they reach number 5, they will be comfortably sated, not eating past the point of fullness. And although reaching number 2 or number 6 is sometimes unavoidable, they need to know that it's best to stay within the range of 3 to 5 if they want to keep their bodies working well.

Here is a demonstration of how to use the scale with children:

1. During a calm, quiet time when there are no distractions, sit down with your child. Talk with her about how important it is for her to keep her body running efficiently (like a well-oiled engine), and remind her that she is the one who has to know how to do this.

2. Show your child the scale. Write it down on a piece of paper and then let her put it into her own words. Depending on the age of the child, use words to help guide her, encouraging her to come up with her own way of describing her hunger. You can also try connecting her degree of hunger to a particular color, if the visual association makes more sense to her.

3. Explain how important it is that her body not go too long without fuel. Describe how she may feel if she lets herself get to a 1 or 2, and tell her that she will need to listen very closely to her body's signals so that she eats when she is at number 3 (hungry).

4. Just as important, teach your child that it's best to stop eating when she reaches number 5 on the scale, and help her to recognize what number 5 feels like. Some

children get into the habit of eating to 6 or 7, which is what can lead to chronic overeating and weight gain. If you are concerned about this, you will have to teach your child how to change what it feels like when she stops eating. Explain that it's dangerous to overfill your engine with gas because it will no longer run efficiently. If you keep reinforcing the idea of staying in the 5-to-3 zone, you will be helping your child to reinforce her connection to her body's signals.

5. Develop a shorthand version of the scale. You can put some key words with associated colors and numbers up on the fridge. Guide your child to look at it—especially if she seems to be asking for extra portions. Make sure she understands that if she is really still hungry, she can certainly have more, but she needs to take a moment to listen to the signal. If it's hard to detect, she will have to wait longer. (More to follow on this in the Waiting Game exercise on page 132.)

6. Help your child think about what her body felt like after she had one helping. Was she still hungry? If she still felt "starved," point out to her that she may have waited too long to eat, which means that it may take more food to fill her up and a longer time for her brain to get the message from her stomach that she was comfortable and could stop.

7. Ask your child what it felt like the last time she ended up eating so much that she felt stuffed. Use words she likes to use and try to engage her curiosity about her body. Ask your child, for example, "Was your stomach so full that it felt like it was going to burst?" Younger children, especially from about age three, love talking

about poop and farts and enjoy laughing about their bodies. Use their and your sense of humor.

8. Help your child understand that keeping track of what her body is telling her can take time, and she should try to be patient. Also, remind her that sometimes it's hard to hear the body's signal, so strengthening the connection between her belly and her head can take a lot of concentration. Help her make the connection between this kind of strengthening and strengthening the muscles that allow her to do the things she loves to do—concentrate on a game with her friend, play at recess, climb the jungle gym, ride her bike, and so on. Use examples that are pertinent to your child's particular interests, and remember—you cannot remind your child enough or reinforce the message too often.

Flexibility Is Key!

OF COURSE, THERE WILL be days and times when your child (or you for that matter!) are at a 1 or a 7. In fact, there are times when you yourself may choose to keep eating to the point of being stuffed because the food is simply divine. The beauty is that if you have good habits overall, you can return to them with confidence. That is why you want to help your children know their own bodies and keep listening to those signals. By keeping the signals loud and clear, they are able to have flexibility in their lives as well as develop good habits that keep them healthy and knowing how to eat for life.

Satiety

All children can learn how to self-regulate and eat in moderation once they tune in to what it feels like to be sated. It's important to remember, however, that the concept of satiety (feeling comfortably full) is both physical and psychological. Have you ever had a full-course meal, couldn't eat another bite, even left some meat and potatoes on your plate, but when dessert was served, you suddenly had room? Often, we want dessert because we are looking for a sense of completion to the meal. Food should be enjoyed, not simply used to fill hunger. We need to help our children learn to enjoy this process as we relearn how to enjoy our own food.

One important element of being able to feel psychologically full is to understand that food is not going away and you will always be able to eat more of a desired food if you want it. Look at young children at a birthday party who have not yet learned that cake is a more desirable food than carrots; they often eat several bites of cake and then are off and running to the next activity. They are not thinking they'd better eat all the cake at once because they will not have the opportunity the next day. They live—and eat—in the moment, staying tuned in to their bodies' signals. And when their body says they are done, they are done.

This idea of access is key for children to understand. If they think food is disappearing and will be out of their reach, then they are going to want to demand more of it— even if they know they are full. In order for a child to pay attention to his body's signals, he needs to know that he will be able to get the food he wants. In addition, giving children access allows them to enjoy the food they are having in the moment, which cuts down on overeating. I have worked with countless compulsive eaters who state that they never even tasted the food they were stuffing down their throats because they always felt they "shouldn't" be eating it. We do not want this to be a habit our children develop. I am a big believer in enjoying the food you eat, every bite of it! Food is to be savored.

Jennifer is one mother who used the Hunger-Fullness scale to help her seven-year-old son, Sammy, begin to reconnect with his body's signals. Sammy is an exuberant and energetic young boy who had always been on the high end of the growth curve for height and weight. Like his father, Jonathan, and his uncles, he is tall and has always had a tendency to gain weight. His parents were not concerned, however, until he hit the age of five, when his mother began to notice that Sammy didn't seem to self-regulate as well as his older brother, who was shorter and lean, and who generally ate until he was full and then stopped.

Sammy's dad had often joked that his own signal of fullness is his clean plate, and that he never feels full until the food is taken away from him! Now Jennifer and Jonathan began to notice that Sammy seemed to have this same tendency, and they didn't want him to battle with a weight problem like his dad and uncles. Jennifer and Jonathan didn't want to approach Sammy in a negative or critical way, but they did want to see whether they could help prevent him from developing problems.

I gave Sammy's parents the Hunger-Fullness scale with instructions and suggested that they present the process as an investigation to engage his curiosity. Since Sammy loved cars, they used the analogy of gas, fuel, and cars to help him connect with the idea of fueling his body. They compared the electrical system that delivers signals from the engine to the "brain" of the car to the signals his tummy delivered to his own brain. They explained to Sammy that some people have a harder time hearing their body's message that they are full, and Sammy might be one of those people whose "whistle" is softer, so he needed to pay closer attention and listen more carefully to his body's messages. Sammy's job was to make sure he was giving his body a chance to hear the whistle's signal. They sat down together, and Sammy helped adapt the scale, giving elaborate descriptions to the numbers. (I will let you fill in the blanks, knowing how much kids love to joke about poop and farts. Sammy was quite a riot coming up with words to describe the gradations of fullness!)

They tacked the scale on the fridge where Sammy could see it and use it to help him figure out what signals his stomach was sending his brain. At mealtimes, whenever he asked for a second or third helping, his mother would respond, "Remember to stop for a moment. Let's give your stomach ten minutes to send the message to your brain so you can hear it loud and clear." Then, while they waited, they would chat about the day's activities, or Sammy would help with an activity in the kitchen. When the time was up, he would look at the scale posted on the fridge. Sometimes he would say, "Well, I am definitely still hungry." When that happened, his mother would congratulate him on hearing the signal clearly, and he would eat more. And when he determined that he was no longer hungry, his mother would give him that same congratulatory response for hearing the signal clearly; he just wouldn't eat more.

At first, Sammy had trouble figuring out when he was perfectly comfortable or sated. But knowing that he could eat more if he wanted, he began gradually to feel more comfortable and confident, and to stop asking for second and third helpings at every meal. The more in tune with his own body he became, the less frequently he continued to eat until he was stuffed. Now he is eating when he is hungry and stopping when he is sated. It's clear that he has reconnected to the signal of satiety that helps him stop when he feels comfortably full, and his parents no longer worry that he will have a weight problem.

The Waiting Game

Another way to teach your children how to pay attention to their satiety signal is by helping them learn how to wait. Waiting will help them to distinguish between really wanting food and wanting something else (attention, comfort, a new activity, and so on). As in the case of Sammy, mentioned above, teaching children to wait requires helping them to understand their own bodies. Again, the principle of access is important: when children trust that food is not being taken away, they learn to pay closer attention to their bodies' signals of hunger and fullness. You can start to do this with children at about age four; with a three-year-old you will probably have to do the distracting yourself. Here's a step-by-step model of how to play the Waiting Game: feel free to adapt it in whatever way works for you and your family.

1. Present the exercise as a game. "Would you like to play a game together?"

2. Make a series of suggestions to help your child decide what to do while she's waiting. Perhaps suggest that she play with her toys, or that you go on an outing together. If you think your child may need to unwind in a different way, suggest taking a rest or reading a book—even watching some television. Shifting her attention may help her relax. You need to use your knowledge of your particular child to tune in to the activity that will work best. I often ask my child who has trouble with transitions if she wants to help me make dinner, empty the dishwasher, or plan the next day's lunch.

3. Explain that because it sometimes takes longer for her belly to send the signal to her head that she is full, you are asking her to wait twenty to thirty minutes to see if she is still hungry.

4. Try getting her to identify what she is feeling. "Are you feeling bored?" "Are you feeling tired?" "Are you feeling sad, lonely, scared about anything?"

5. Return to the idea that sometimes we think we still want to eat, but it is not because we are hungry and need the food. Remind her that the food is always there, and that in a half hour, if she is still hungry she can eat. Begin to teach her the notion of feeling fullness in the belly, yet also recognize her desire to have a sweet for its pleasurable taste at the end of the meal. You can reinforce the idea that it's important to eat some food that will help her brain and muscles feel good, not just her mouth and tongue (sugar). Explain

that it is preferable to fill up on nutritious foods, so it is important for her to listen closely to what her body is telling her it is wanting: Is her stomach still hungry, or is it just the desire for another taste in her mouth to feel sated? If you continue to reinforce this information about why we want to eat various foods, including sweets, your child will be less likely to overeat sweets and set up a power struggle with you. Always remind her that she can have the sweet at another time if she determines she doesn't need it now.

If at the end of the specified time period, your child is still demanding another slice of pizza, for example, it's crucial that you follow through and allow your child to have the pizza—even if this feels uncomfortable for you. By showing your child that you respect her decision, you are reinforcing the idea that she is in charge of her own body.

Taking Care of Their Bodies

The more you help your children pay attention to their signals of hunger and fullness, the more you increase their motivation to take care of their bodies and feed them well. Patty came to me because her six-year-old daughter, Lesley, was demanding food nonstop from the minute she picked her up from school, and it was driving her crazy. Not only did Patty not want to stop for a snack or keep preparing food nonstop from 3 until 8 P.M., but she also worried that her daughter, who was in the hundredth percentile for weight and height, would become overweight.

Step Two: Reboot the Connection Between the Belly and the Head

When we examined Lesley's eating pattern, it became clear that she was not a child who was very hungry when she first awakened in the morning. Then, as the day wore on, the distractions of school kept her mind off her hunger. She rarely ate lunch, so by the end of school at 3 P.M. she had eaten almost nothing all day and was quite naturally "starving"—a number 1 on the Hunger-Fullness scale, which is very difficult to recover from. While some children's bodies and metabolism can handle this degree of hunger, Lesley's couldn't, which was why she was so voraciously starving after school and unable to fill herself up.

This was clearly a child who was not listening to the more subtle signs of hunger her body was sending and who was letting herself become so ravenous that it then took much longer and much more food for her body to send the signal to her brain that she was full. Patty began to engage her in the idea of taking care of her body. This appealed to Lesley, since she was very interested in medical matters, even at the tender age of seven. Her mother reminded her that she was the one responsible for her body because she would know best what her body needed. Patty then showed her the Hunger-Fullness scale, which Lesley adapted into a color chart, even remarking that it was more like a circle, a discovery that sparked her curiosity.

In the morning, when Lesley was not that hungry, Patty was able to remind her about how starving she would feel after school, and to suggest that she might want to take something to eat along the way so that she never reached a 1 or 2 degree of hunger.

Together Patty and I discussed the fact that this particular child needed real food as her after-school snack, and that it would be worthwhile for her to sit down to a meal rather than wait for dinner. Patty encouraged her to sit down for soup and a sandwich if she continued to be famished after school. Then, at dinner, if all she wanted was a small portion of what everyone else was eating, her mother would feel comfortable being flexible. As Patty continued to experiment with these ideas, Lesley did take on more responsibility and began to pay more attention to her more subtle signals of hunger. She did begin eating a more substantial snack after school, and as a result, she no longer needed to demand food incessantly between three and eight o'clock.

"*You Are the Expert*"

Eating is a biologically driven process, and yet, culturally, we seem driven to establish some order around feeding rather than simply eating when we are hungry. These attempts at scheduling meals can, however, interfere with a child's natural eating schedule. Indeed, like adults, some children can go for very long periods of time without eating, while others need to eat every few hours. Some kids must start the day with breakfast while others are not hungry until several hours after rising. When children become hungry varies from one individual to the next, and it's usually better to find out what suits your child's body, rather than to try to make his or her body fit into a preestablished routine.

One aspect of respecting kids' individual body needs is helping them learn how to eat for themselves—not to please a parent or caregiver. Kids thrive on your respect for their decisions, and there is no more concrete way to show them that respect than by allowing them to make a decision about whether they are hungry or full. Doing that reinforces the message that they—not you—are the experts on their bodies, and the better they understand that, the more they will trust in and listen to their bodies' signals and begin to derive satisfaction from their ability to take care of their bodies. I always say to kids, "You are the expert on your body; nobody but you knows how hungry or full you are, or what kind of food your body is telling you it wants. You get that information from your tummy. I can't know it. So you have to pay attention and listen to it."

While it might be worthwhile to give a child a chance to eat more if she appears distracted, let us think about the message we are communicating if we encourage our children to "eat one more bite for Mommy (or Daddy)" on an ongoing basis. First, we are communicating to the child that he does not understand his own body's signals and that he needs to disregard these signals. Second, we are teaching him that eating involves a feeling in his belly past the point of comfort (number 6 or 7 on the hunger chart). Remember, it is eating to the point beyond fullness or until stuffed on a chronic basis that promotes weight gain. And third, we are communicating that he should eat for reasons other than the signals he is getting from his belly.

If you worry that your children are not eating enough because they are picky or small eaters and you keep encouraging them to eat more, they may begin to eat more to please you, so that you worry less and feel better as parents. Conversely, parents can be too critical and overinvolved by making such comments as, "Haven't you had enough? Aren't you full now? You don't really need that." Such remarks undermine children's confidence in knowing their bodies just as much as urging them to eat more, and they can trigger a silent rebellion manifested by covert eating and weight gain, despite any overt attempts at weight control.

If your goal as a parent is to help your children make their own decisions, it is vitally important that you also help them stay connected to their own cues. If your child is temperamentally easygoing and compliant, he will be more likely to follow your cues than his own, and such compliance can make it difficult for a parent to determine if the child is listening to his belly or listening to his mom and dad. Ironically, children who are strong-willed and have a more intense temperament, while they may protest more and create more of a fight with food, also tend to be the ones who pay more attention to their own signals of hunger and fullness and defend their ownership of their own bodies.

A Quick Review

It's up to parents to teach children to eat when they are hungry, to pay attention to those signals, and to stop when they are full. Encourage them to develop good eating habits and eat a rich variety of foods, then model that behavior. I laugh when my two older daughters say to their youngest sister (who, as I've stated, is a very picky eater and doesn't like to eat very much), "Great! May we have your carrots?" My youngest daughter then becomes very possessive of that food because she sees it is the desired item, and more often than not she decides to eat it herself. If you don't try to push food onto (or into) a child, she will often come around.

Here are the crucial messages to communicate continually to your children:

- You are the expert on your own body.
- Nobody but you knows when you are hungry or full and what that feels like.
- You need to listen to your body and make sure you pay attention to the messages/signals it is giving you, even when those signals come in a soft voice.

The more you can help your children pay attention to and respect these signals the more your children will feel you respect them, which will, in turn, help build their self-respect.

Now that you have worked with your children on Steps One and Two, talking to them about nutrition and helping them reconnect to their bodies' signals of hunger and fullness, you should be starting to see some changes in their eating behavior. With that in mind, let me ask you a few questions:

- Does your child seem to struggle less around mealtime?
- Does she have less trouble transitioning or decelerating from one activity to another?

- Is your child becoming more adept at picking up her body's signal that she is hungry or full?

- Are you more comfortable with giving your child fuller access to all foods?

- Are you less worried that your child is eating too much or too little?

- Are you more comfortable letting him decide how much or how little of a meal he wants to eat?

- Are you able to give your child a choice and then remind her the next day that this was the choice she made?

- Has your child begun to see the consequences of these choices?

- Have you then used this cause-and-effect as a way to guide her to make a different choice the next day?

If you answered yes to even one of the above questions, you should feel reassured and encouraged that your children are learning how to pay attention to their signals of hunger and fullness. As they learn to tune in to their bodies, their confidence will grow, and your worries will lessen. Kids can and will learn to eat when they are hungry and stop when they are full. Parents simply need to give them some tools that will allow them to pay attention to and develop a sense of responsibility toward their bodies.

In the next chapter, you will see how to build further on this connection by helping your children distinguish their feelings of hunger from other feelings.

CHAPTER SIX

Step Three: Separate Hunger and Fullness from Other Feelings

M OST ADULTS UNDERSTAND what it is to eat
for emotional reasons. We can all think of times
when we've turned to food to assuage difficult
feelings such as anxiety, fatigue, loneliness, or distress. But
many of us are still surprised to hear that children as young
as five or six might also begin to use food to soothe their
emotions. We like to think of children as being happy and
carefree all the time. As parents, it is difficult for us to accept the fact that our children may not always feel confident or good about themselves, or that they might struggle
at times and feel sad or frustrated. Even more difficult for
us to accept is the idea that we cannot always solve or fix
our children's problems.

In this chapter, we will look at how children can use
food for emotional reasons, which can create eating problems for them. We will also look at three simple ways to
help kids learn to identify their emotions so they can then
separate those feelings from hunger. Once they can do this,

children are more likely to stay connected to their signals of hunger and fullness, to eat moderately, and not to turn to food as a way to comfort themselves.

When Kids Use Food for Soothing, Control, or Distraction

When kids begin to eat for emotional reasons, they are more than likely reaching for food as a way to calm themselves and "eat" their feelings instead of experiencing them. And parents can unwittingly encourage this behavior. I think all parents will acknowledge that food can be a great pacifier. Haven't we all on occasion reached for a cookie to distract or soothe our upset child? Or sent food to the backseat of the car in response to the old, annoying "Are we there yet?"

Using food to distract a child or alleviate his boredom from time to time will not create a problem, but it is critical that children not use food habitually for these purposes. Since food is the first tangible arena in which kids can exert control, they often use mealtimes, as well as their parents' agendas with regard to diet and nutrition, to act or play out other emotional issues. Additionally, children can quickly learn to use food, which is stimulating to the mouth and the taste buds, to soothe or distract themselves. For all these reasons, it becomes very important for them to figure out how to identify their feelings and to differentiate emotions from hunger. Once children become more familiar with their myriad emotions—from boredom to anger to sadness or loneliness—the less likely they will be to turn to food to soothe themselves. In fact, they will be learning two important skills at once:

1. How to deal with their feelings
2. How to stay in touch with their hunger

Indeed, knowing what they feel is a way for children to begin making confident decisions. (Step Four in the next chapter.)

Don't Try to Fix Their Feelings

In order to navigate life, one of the skills all children need is the ability to handle or manage the intensity of their feelings. If they think their parents are there to assuage or get rid of their feelings, children will never learn to deal with their powerful emotions. We know that when small children are overwhelmed by their emotions, they can have temper tantrums. Tantrums are a way of acting out the fact that they cannot manage their emotions, and for small children such reactions are age appropriate. Young children also turn to food as a means of control, because food is one of the first things they can control—no one can force a child to eat if he doesn't want to. If parents are not skilled at seeing how the fights their children create around food are often their only way of communicating, small children can end up manipulating an entire family. We want our children to be able to assert their needs by communicating verbally; we want them to be able to talk about their feelings so that we understand what they need from us. We do not want them to turn to food to soothe or comfort themselves if they are not getting their needs understood or met. But how do we teach them how to verbalize their feelings, or even how to separate the food fight in which they are engaging us from what they are really feeling? Children do not necessarily need us to fix their problems, but at times they do need us to help them identify what they are feeling.

Eileen was struggling to face the fact that her seven-year-old daughter, Polly, had begun to use food to help herself feel better. "It is so painful," she said, with some anguish in her voice, "to imagine that Polly may be feeling bad about herself. For the last year, I've noticed that she always asks for extra helpings, and I'm beginning to conclude that this is because she's unhappy at times.

"We've always tried to make her feel so loved and let her know how great we think she is. I can't imagine why she would be feeling bad about herself. But she does at times say these things, and I think I have to stop ignoring them. I also think she has been using those extra helpings of ice cream or mac and cheese to help herself feel better."

Although Polly was trying to let her parents know how she was feeling, she was at an age when it was difficult for her to verbalize her feelings directly. Once Eileen began to tune in and realize that it was hard for her to see Polly in distress, she was able to provide her daughter with a way to talk about some of the things that were making her feel bad at school.

"When Polly asked for a second helping of dessert," Eileen said, "I would ask her what had happened at school that day. Then Polly started to tell me that on some days her best friend ignored her. We began to talk about how this made her feel. The amazing thing was that after a while, she was able to tell me directly when her feelings had been hurt. After she began to be able to tell me she felt bad, she stopped asking for those second and third helpings. Now when she complains that she's hungry or bored, I figure out ways for her to tell me more about what's going on. Since I've learned to give her room to talk about these feelings, she has actually started to feel more confident about figuring out what to do and is asserting herself more with her friends! This doesn't make every day a happy day, but I am amazed by how well she's learned to calm down in other ways. And I'm a lot more confident, too. I don't get so worried when I see she's had a bad day."

Polly and Eileen's situation is very common but not so

Red Flags

IF YOU ARE WONDERING whether or not your children may be eating for emotional reasons, consider this list of red flags:

- They fight about food fairly frequently: "I want another ice pop! I need another ice pop!"
- They are asking for more and more helpings and don't seem to want to take a breath in between.
- They complain a lot about being bored, and when they do, you notice them diving into their food.
- They have a sad look on their face but are unable to describe what they are feeling. When they eat, they seem happier.

complicated to address. Through the process of Eileen's tuning in to her daughter and helping her to understand her own emotions, Eileen was able to help Polly find ways other than food to soothe her hurt feelings. And once Polly identified and validated her feelings, she was able to separate those feelings from hunger. It's crucial, however, that parents become involved in helping kids to identify and process their emotions, so that they aren't over-whelmed by them.

Help Your Kids Understand Their Feelings

Our children need to know that it's okay for them to feel however they feel. Our kids also need to know that we can handle the fact that they can have feelings that are not al-ways so "pretty" or "nice." As their parent, you are in the best position to help your children begin to recognize and label their feelings. By taking a moment to tune in and think about (or intuit) what they may be feeling, you can begin to give them the language they need to understand and identify their experience.

Children don't automatically know how to put feelings into words; it is a process they are learning, and you are teaching them. It's up to you to help them identify not only their feelings but also the connection between how they feel and what's going on in their lives. Knowing their per-sonalities and paying attention to their day-to-day lives, you can begin to see and then suggest how they might be feeling and why. Then you can prompt them with the ap-propriate words. They will get better and better at this, and being able to express their feelings will become a way to soothe themselves. It helps them make sense of their inner experience, and it helps them feel that their feelings are valid. Often, in fact, it is this process in and of itself that enables them to stop using food emotionally.

A Quick Exercise

1. Observe your child's face. Take a moment to really see him. Try to identify your own feelings and then separate them from those of your child.

2. Based on your observation, suggest how your child may be feeling. "You are looking like you are feeling sad. Is that true?" "Are you worried, frightened, hurt, or angry?"

3. Take a moment to see how he reacts. If he denies the feeling, you can say, "Hmm, it just seemed like something was upsetting to you. Tell me what you were just doing." This sometimes helps a child connect to the event, and also helps you to empathize and imagine what he might have felt. You can then validate his feelings further by saying something such as, "Hmm, if that had happened to me, I might feel pretty angry (sad, etc.)." Give him a moment and some space to see if he is understanding what you are saying. Sometimes you can tell by a child's face that you have accurately identified what he is feeling—even if he doesn't want to admit it. In this case, a simple hug will often do. He knows that you know, and that is very comforting.

4. Try to ask specific questions that give context to your child's feelings. At times, especially if they are young,

children tend to respond vaguely to open-ended questions. "You look a bit sad. What did you do at recess today? Who did you play with?"

5. Explain that it is sometimes hard to know what exactly he is feeling. Feelings can be disguised. For example, anger sometimes comes from frustration and disappointment.

6. Try to help him differentiate one feeling from another. "Sometimes it's hard to know if you are really angry because you're frustrated that you can't read that chapter book very well. Are you feeling disappointed or frustrated with yourself?"

7. Help the child connect certain events in his life to his emotions. For example, you might say, "Do you feel angry when Tommy doesn't play with you? Does that hurt your feelings? Do you end up feeling sad or frustrated?" "I know you really wanted to sing that part in chorus; it can be disappointing when we don't get what we want. How are you doing with this?"

Young children have difficulty putting their feelings into language, not only because they don't have the words yet but also because the feelings themselves can be overwhelming, and they don't yet have the ability to differentiate one from another. By doing these exercises with them, you will help them not only to develop the language but also to distinguish between, for example, feelings of anger and sadness. Here are a few more tips for helping very young children (ages one to three) who have less ability to express their feelings:

- When your child says "I'm hungry" and you suspect she may actually not be hungry, give her a piece of paper and some crayons. Ask her to draw what she might be feeling inside her body. You might be surprised by what you see!

- Ask her about the drawing: "What made you think of using that color? What could the little girl be thinking or feeling? Can you tell me about your drawing?" Young children represent themselves in other objects or people; you can say things such as, "That sun you drew is so red! How does the sun feel (or the house, or the grass): Happy? Sad?" Or, "That little boy looks so mad! What is he feeling? What just happened to him?"

The more tools your children have to differentiate among their emotions, the closer they will stay connected to their bodies and the gradations of hunger and fullness. Equally important, by teaching them these skills you will be allowing them to feel understood and you will also be communicating a message: "It is okay to feel what you are feeling." By doing that, you give them an opportunity to process feelings that can be difficult, including jealousy, anger, competitiveness, disappointment, frustration, sadness, anxiety, and confusion, to name but a few. I cannot emphasize enough how important it is to help children process their feelings. In the fifteen years I have been treating people of all ages with all sorts of food disorders, I've found that one of the key issues is their use of food to process their emotions—to soothe, to distract, and to control. By helping your children to know and remain connected to their emotional world and to communicate their feelings, you are giving them one of the most powerful tools they can have to prevent them from developing life-long problems with food.

Boredom Is a Good Teacher

Children often complain of being bored and may begin to confuse their boredom with hunger. My response whenever I hear a child say she is bored is, "Great! What a wonderful opportunity for you to sit quietly and be with yourself; let's see where you go from there."

Often, and especially with young children, complaints of boredom signal their needing or wanting your attention. If you realize this is the case, try to focus on your child for a moment and tell her, "I'll be right with you after I finish this phone call," or "Let's sit together after I finish with this paperwork; I promise I won't forget!"

If you are able to drop what you're doing at that moment, great, but children need to learn how to wait, and the best way for them to learn that is if they know you will be there as soon as you are able. This is similar to teaching them the Waiting Game (page 132), in which you helped them wait for their heads to get the message that their bellies are full. Again, it's key to reinforce the idea of access. If your children know they will have your attention in a few moments (or a few hours if they are older), it will be easier for them to WAIT. The ability to wait is one of the most important psychological tools your children can develop; it helps in delaying gratification, which will reward them in all sorts of ways, and, of course, gives them the capacity to stay tuned in to their signals of hunger and fullness.

If your child complains of boredom, it is your job as the parent not to dissuade her from what she is feeling, but rather to help her get to know her feelings more intimately. Consider the following dialogue:

Parent: "So, you feel bored. Great! Now you have a chance to discover something about yourself. Take a bit of time to just sit. Notice what you start to think about. What do you notice about how you feel? What might you think to do about this feeling?"

Again, you do not want to jump in and try to fix her boredom for her. She needs the space to go inside herself and discover what it is she is feeling. Even if she is asking (or demanding!) that you do so, try to resist the impulse and encourage her to deal with the emotional situation on her own terms.

Children can learn to tolerate their own boredom. In a quiet space with nothing to do, children are freed from distractions and can begin to examine their inner experience. Too often, our children do not know themselves, and that is partly because they can be so overstimulated that they become reliant on external stimulation. When children learn to identify their emotional states accurately, they are more likely to stay in touch with their inner states of hunger, fullness, fatigue, or level of energy; it is this connection to their body that, if maintained, helps prevent disordered eating.

Most often, children are quite creative and have a wealth of ideas with which to engage themselves—if parents get out of the way. Getting out of our children's way can be difficult because we often feel it is our job to stimulate them. If that's what we believe, however, we are likely to miss an important point, which is that children are very good at discovering the world and stimulating themselves. Young children, particularly babies and toddlers, often get so involved in their worlds that they are never bored.

By giving your children the space to be bored, you will help them tolerate this state of mind long enough to discover and use their imaginations without communicating the idea that boredom is something that needs to be fixed with food.

Power Struggles Can Signal Emotional Distress

If they feel life is confusing or out of control, children will frequently seize on the one thing over which they can feel some sense of power: food!

Kenny was a single father who talked with me about his son Ronald. Ronald had just turned four when Kenny began to notice him turning mealtimes into power struggles. Kenny had no idea how to handle the situation and stated that when he was growing up, "We just ate. We never even thought about it, much less fought about it!"

Preoccupied with other issues (he had also begun to care for his own mother, who was ill at the time), Kenny hadn't imagined that Ronald's fights about food could possibly have any connection with how he might be feeling. Because food had always been very straightforward for Kenny, he never imagined that the fights Ronald was creating at dinner had to do with anything other than food. As he began to talk more directly with Ronald about the changes in their lives, he made a point of explaining that he was aware that they were spending less time together and certainly would understand if Ronald were feeling bad about this. Ronald then began to behave less aggressively at mealtimes, and Kenny, in turn, began to give him a bit more control over what he ate and when he had his desserts. In a couple of weeks, Kenny noticed that dinnertime had become less tense. Additionally, Ronald began to talk with him about missing some of the time they used to have together. In talking about the issues and getting out of the fight with food, they figured out some solutions to adapt to the changing needs of the family.

The important thing here is to be able to separate one issue from another: Is your child using food to communicate another feeling? Is he reacting to some change in his environment? It is sometimes very easy for parents to get involved in discussing the food itself and thus reinforcing the struggle. But simply by recognizing, validating, and helping kids identify their feelings, we can help them avoid feeling overwhelmed or out of control.

And although we are concerned here specifically about eating behavior, when we help our children to recognize and differentiate among their feelings, we are teaching them to manage their emotions in general. By helping kids get in touch with how they feel and not avoid feelings that are painful, we are teaching them that:

1. They can figure out what they are feeling;
2. What they are feeling is okay;

3. Although some feelings are scary or hard, having the feeling is not the end of the world; and
4. Feelings are normal and they can live through them. Feelings are part of life.

The exercise that follows provides both you and your children with a useful tool for practicing how to manage intense feelings.

The Wave Exercise

The Wave Exercise helps teach children about the nature of emotions and how to manage those feelings. Specifically, it can help children see how emotions and feelings first gain in intensity and then die down. This exercise shows children how to identify their feelings and to not always say they are hungry when a big emotion seems to overwhelm them. It can also help them to learn how to self-soothe as they figure out other ways to calm or comfort themselves—regardless of their age. By learning how to hold on to their emotions, they will learn to wait out the intensity and not try to assuage an emotional need with food. Once they tune in to their own emotions, their need to develop ways to distance themselves from them and soothe themselves (via food, drugs, etc.) naturally decreases.

1. Describe a wave. Then explain how feelings are exactly like waves: they build up and then they die down. Here is an example: "Remember how angry you were feeling when I said you couldn't watch any more TV? That feeling inside when it was at its strongest was like the

biggest and highest part of the wave. But it died down after a while—maybe after an hour or the next day. It didn't stay as powerful or as big forever."

2. Using a scale of 1 to 10, explain how the intensity of different feelings can change from high to low. Explain how, when they may feel very, very angry, their feeling would be a 10. If they feel only a little sad, their feeling would be a 2 or 3.

3. If children have difficulty labeling their feelings, try to guide them. Tuned-in parents can often intuit their children's feelings or moods and can label the feeling for them—especially for younger children.

4. Ask your children to remember the last time they had an intense feeling. Then ask them if that feeling became less intense after some time had passed—an hour or a day, for example.

5. When they are having negative feelings, offer them reassurance or comfort. Perhaps they will allow you to hug them and talk about it. Or perhaps you will need to wait until the intensity of the emotion, particularly anger, dies down to a 3 before they allow you to hold them and comfort them.

6. If they try to avoid the feeling, or go around it, they might get stuck in it. Explain that trying to avoid a negative feeling often makes it more intense. Help them understand that in the middle of an intense feeling (a 10), it is very hard to figure out a solution. However, once that feeling dies down to maybe a 2 or 3, or even a 4, they will feel more capable of figuring out what to do.

7. Above all, try to listen to your kids and not jump in to try to fix the feeling. By allowing them to feel the feel-

ing, you are teaching your children that feelings are not dangerous and are not facts—they change and go away.

8. Once they begin to calm down and either accept your soothing or learn to soothe themselves, they will be able to understand the scenario or situation that precipitated the emotion. By learning to link the situation to the resulting emotion, they will be able to feel their feelings instead of using food to block or avoid them. And very important, once the intensity of the feeling dies down, you can begin to solve problems together during a calmer, more rational moment.

Keep remembering that you want to help your child learn about his feelings, but you also need to set limits on acting out, such as tantrums, whining, badgering, and so on. You can always talk together to validate the child's feelings after he has calmed down.

Becoming a Body Detective, or What Does Hunger FEEL Like?

Before you decide your child is eating emotionally, you always want to rule out the possibility that he is truly hungry. It is quite common for children to be ravenous for several days or even weeks before a growth spurt. Remember how infants eat every hour or two just before those growth spurts? They are actually pumping up your milk production so there will be enough when their bodies need it!

The Hunger Exercise

When your child says "I'm hungry!" over and over again, you can create a dialogue that goes something like this:

1. "You keep saying you're hungry, and maybe you are; let's figure this out. Close your eyes and tell me where the hunger is in your body. Is it in your head? Is it in your stomach? Is it in your arms and legs?"

2. "What does it feel like? Is it an ache? A feeling of gnawing or emptiness?" If the feeling occurs anywhere but in the stomach, state the following: "Hunger is always felt in your stomach first. If you are having this feeling in another part of your body, your body is trying to tell you something else. Let's try to figure out what your body is saying you need. Is it a hug? Do you want to play a game with me?"

3. Help your child further identify the feeling. "Could you be feeling worried or upset about something? Angry? Confused? Nervous? Sometimes these feelings happen and we think that we are hungry instead."

4. Explain that sometimes it's hard to figure out if we need to eat because we are hungry or because we need something else, but be sure to reassure him that food is always available.

5. If your child insists he is feeling the hunger in his belly and he therefore still wants dessert, remind him that dessert is the fun food and it is best to fill his belly with other kinds of food first. Remind him that he can still have dessert and again that the food is always available. If he has already had his treat for the day, remind him that he can have the chips, cookies, or candy he's asking for tomorrow.

When Kids Are Tired

WHEN KIDS ARE TIRED, they frequently think they are hungry. And since children tend to resist ever admitting they are tired, they will do almost anything to avoid slowing down and taking a rest. Try to figure out for yourself if this might be the case (especially with younger children, up until about age seven). Help the child do an activity that is calming and restful and see whether he slows down. Whether or not he was tired, doing that will help him calm down so that he may be more receptive to showing you his feelings, because the connection will be clearer to him and more evident to you.

A Quick Review

Here are some key points to remember about teaching your kids to separate hunger from their other feelings:

1. You are strengthening your children's connection to their emotions as well as the connection between their stomachs and their brains.
2. You are giving them the ability to take the time and develop the language with which to describe and then communicate their feelings.
3. You are validating their feelings for them.
4. You are giving them the tools they need to be able to soothe themselves in the face of strong emotions and helping them to avoid using food (drugs, etc.) to achieve that end.

5. You are building their ability to be less afraid of and intimidated by strong emotions as well as their ability to manage strong feelings.

6. You are helping them to see that you as their parents are not scared or intimidated by their having strong feelings; this increases their feelings of safety and comfort and decreases their need to cover things up or stuff down their feelings because they don't want to worry you.

7. You are teaching them that feelings are a part of life.

8. You are building problem-solving skills by helping them learn how to wait until after the intensity of the emotion dies down in order to figure out solutions. You are not invalidating their emotions but instead teaching them how to incorporate both the emotional and the rational into the thinking process.

By accomplishing these goals, you are decreasing the likelihood that your children will turn to food to soothe, solve, or distract themselves from emotions. As your children begin to manage their feelings and keep them separate from hunger, they will be laying the groundwork for becoming good decision makers. In the next chapter, you will see how your kids can use the tools they've acquired for understanding their feelings to make rational, thoughtful decisions about food.

CHAPTER SEVEN

Step Four: Teach Your Child to Become a Confident Decision Maker

A parent who continually picks up the pieces becomes a feedback system which prevents a youngster from developing one of her own. Unfortunately, it is sometimes necessary to tie yourself to the sofa and let a child feel the effects of her own carelessness.

JANE M. HEALY, PH.D.,
YOUR CHILD'S GROWING MIND

The other day in the grocery line, my daughter asked if she could have one of those treats they always have there. I responded: "Well, what do you think? You know how to make that decision." And she responded: "Actually, I don't think I want it now." The lady behind me with her two-year-old just about fell over and said: "How on earth did you do that?"

MOTHER OF AN EIGHT-YEAR-OLD GIRL

A PRIME GOAL for all parents is to help teach their children how to make decisions confidently and responsibly. How do we make our kids confident decision makers? We keep them safe, give them choices, encourage decision making, and support them, regardless of the outcome and without rescuing them from the consequences. In Step Three, you focused on helping your children learn more about their emotions in order to prevent them from getting into the habit of using food for emotional purposes. In Step Four, children are going to use this knowledge to learn how to become confident decision makers who are able to make food choices and understand the consequences of those choices.

Decision making involves several steps:

1. Thinking of a choice or decision, and reviewing the either/ors.
2. Thinking through the consequences of each choice.
3. Figuring out how they will feel given the various consequences.

Once children have integrated Steps One through Three (the nutritional information they need to know, the connection to their body's signals of hunger and fullness, and their ability to distinguish hunger from other feelings), they will have cleared the way to making decisions about their food. They can look at a bag of popcorn or an apple and go through an internal dialogue that leads them to a decision about what to eat. Obviously, this will take practice, and we as parents will need to guide them by providing them with both the encouragement and the freedom to make food choices within the parameters we set.

The rewards for doing this are enormous: the fight is taken out of food, we are no longer food cops with treats, and we can be assured that our children are making healthy decisions for themselves, building confidence, and developing self-respect as they feel our respect for them grow.

When you begin to help your children learn this process, it's important that you take these steps:

1. Establish clear guidelines and parameters with relation to food so your children will feel safe and have some framework within which to make their decisions.
2. Suggest possible outcomes of their choices and decisions.
3. Offer other choices as a way to help them think through their decisions.
4. Validate or help them manage the consequences of the decisions they do make.

In the following pages, you will be learning some specific tools for giving your kids the building blocks they need to make decisions about food.

What Is a Confident Decision Maker?

Before you turn to your children, you might need to start this process by asking yourself: How do I make decisions about food? What might give my child confidence (or give me confidence) in his ability to make these kinds of decisions? Let's take a fairly simple example. Everyone on the planet sometimes eats for emotional reasons. Even if this is not something you do habitually, there are surely those days when nothing will satisfy but that bag of potato chips or box of chocolates. On those days, what do you say to yourself? "I know I'm eating because I'm very nervous about that presentation coming up, but I also know that if I don't eat the chocolates, I'll eat everything else in sight and then eat the chocolates anyway, which will end up making me feel even worse." Or you might say to yourself: "I know myself, and I know that if I eat those chocolates I will end up feeling even worse and I won't be able to move on. I would be better off just taking a brisk walk, or a bath, or calling a friend to vent."

There are no "shoulds" in learning how to make decisions. Whatever your decision, it is important to try to figure out how you might respond, and what the consequences would be. The only way to do that is through trial and error, which enables you to learn more about yourself as you build reference points that predict how you will feel after making a particular decision.

Once you make the choice, you live with it. You will always learn from the result. Perhaps you learn that, more often than not, you feel better when you allow yourself those chocolates because you feel satisfied, and are therefore able to move on. Or you learn that eating them doesn't feel satisfying, so you know that the next time it would be better to take a walk or talk with a friend to distract yourself. Again, there is no right or wrong.

The clearer parents are about how they make decisions for themselves, the more helpful they can be as guides for their children. The more opportunities your children have to test their decisions, the more their confidence and self-respect will develop. That's why it is so important to give them the room they need to try out their own decisions and not to rescue them from the consequences. If we let them sort through their choices and the possible consequences, they will begin to build a data bank of information about themselves so that they can predict how they will feel given a particular outcome in the future.

As they build those reference points, they will be able to make sounder, more thoughtful decisions. For example, they might say, after deciding to have their dessert at breakfast, "Well, I did feel worse not having dessert with my family because I chose to have it for breakfast instead; today I will wait." Parents can help reinforce this connection between their choices and consequences by reminding them, "Remember how you felt when you didn't eat dinner last night and then were so hungry right before bed? Are you going to want to feel that way again tonight, or do you want to have something to eat right before I close the kitchen?"

One important component of this parental clarity is establishing clear parameters for you to refer to and kids to follow.

Establishing Clear Parameters

Before we can help our children learn how to make confident choices and deal with the consequences of those choices, we need to be clear about the parameters we feel safe setting up about food and eating. Once we've done that, we can teach our children how to think through the way they might feel, holding their hands as they begin to learn from the consequences of their decisions and encouraging them to make a new choice the next time. Consider how this process can play out.

Jack, a father with whom I recently worked, was worried because his five-year-old son, Josh, was often not hungry at dinnertime but would always want to eat right before his bedtime. (Of course, after he had brushed his teeth, too!) Jack wasn't comfortable sending Josh to bed hungry, but he was also beginning to resent Josh's stalling at bedtime, and to feel that he and his wife were being held hostage in the kitchen, as mealtimes never seemed to end. (Kids are such experts at bedtime stalling that a friend of mine calls it Bed, Bath and Beyond!)

It's Okay to Go to Bed Hungry

PARENTS NEED NOT worry about sending their children to bed hungry. Believe me, it will not harm them, and they will have enough food to eat the next day. You are not using it as a punishment; you are using what they are telling you to help them take responsibility for their choices. What you are giving them is invaluable: the ability to listen to their bodies and their feelings and then predict how the choices they make cause them to feel.

As I began working with Jack, I suggested that he might be more susceptible to his son's protestations of hunger before bed because Josh was small for his age and a picky eater. I then tried to reassure him that he could be firm in his parameters because if his son did go to bed hungry, he would more than likely eat more the next day. I recommended that Jack and his wife present two choices and let Josh decide which he might prefer:

1. He could eat when he was not very hungry to make sure he would not be hungry right before bed when the kitchen was "closed" (something I encourage all parents to do, so that they are not held hostage in the kitchen).

2. Or, he could not eat as much when he was not hungry, go to bed a little hungrier, and see what that felt like. Perhaps then he would want to eat more the next day.

I predicted that Josh would choose the second option and then complain to the hilt that he was "starving" later on. I warned Jack that this potential reaction from his son would require him to remain firm about the kitchen's being closed. Sure enough, that night Josh chose not to eat and then complained loudly about being hungry. His parents gently reminded him of the choice he had made and suggested that he might end up making a different choice the next day. They walked away when he continued to complain, and when he whined "I'm starved!" as he went to sleep, they replied in a matter-of-fact way: "I guess you will eat more tomorrow, then. As soon as you wake up, you can eat a big breakfast if you are still starving!"

I congratulated these parents on their ability to remain calm in the face of such rigorous complaints. It's so easy to fall for our little ones' cries of hunger. Within a couple of nights, Josh stopped asking for food right before bedtime, and when he sometimes refused dinner, his parents gently reminded him of the hour he had left to eat before the kitchen closed. More often than not, he would then eat a bit, and his attempts to use food in order to postpone bedtime eventually stopped.

Remember, you want to help your child build a data bank of information about his reactions and experiences so that he has some reference points and is able to learn from the choices he makes and their consequences. Even if he resists it at first, he will secretly feel proud of making his own decisions and about the fact that you respect him enough to allow him to do that—even if he doesn't like the outcome. By letting your child go to bed hungry, you are not endangering him. You are giving him the opportunity to discover something about himself.

Keeping Parameters Clear

We as parents need to lay out the consequences of the different decisions our children might make within parameters that are sensible to us and fit within our parenting style. In general, we are trying to reinforce their knowledge of nutrition in order to give them some options and guide them toward being able to weigh the outcomes of various choices. You might, for example, teach a younger child to ask herself, "If I eat three lollipops, will I have enough energy to play with my Legos?" A preadolescent, on the other hand, might be able to make the food-effect connection at a higher cognitive level with a question such as, "If I eat potato chips for dinner, will I end up feeling lousy and angry at myself? If I eat them after dinner, will I feel less hungry and therefore be less prone to eat too many? If I don't eat the potato chips at all, will I feel so deprived that I wind up eating everything else in sight and then have the chips anyway?"

What you should be striving for is a balance between your own comfort zone and your child's freedom to choose. The next story illustrates how a parent figured out how to establish her own parameters and also help her child learn through the consequences of her decisions about food.

Anna is a very precocious seven-year-old who, at the age of six, decided she wanted to become a vegetarian, not only because she (like many young children) hated the taste of meat, but also because she was very interested in animals and truly couldn't bear the thought of eating one. The problem was that Anna was a very picky eater and wouldn't eat any meatless source of protein. As her mother, Molly, struggled to find foods with protein that Anna would eat, their battles over food were becoming quite intense. Molly didn't want to say "No, you can't be a vegetarian," but she couldn't let Anna eat in a way that was not going to be healthy for her. Because she didn't want to deny her daughter's independence and thoughtfulness, she was determined to figure out a way to present her parameters and, at the same time, help her daughter come to her own decision.

In our work together, I helped Molly clarify those parameters.

1. If Anna wanted to take responsibility for her food choices by becoming a vegetarian, she would also have to take responsibility for her body in a respectful, healthy way. This was the bottom line. If she wanted this choice, then she had to deal with the negative consequences of eating some foods she might not like in

order to have the positive consequence of being a vegetarian.

2. If she could not find any other options for protein, she would be unable to make the choice to be a vegetarian.

Once Molly was comfortable setting these limits, Anna felt she was making the decision for herself. And, in fact, she continued to be a vegetarian, began to expand her repertoire of foods, and enjoyed the satisfaction of taking good care of her body. As a bonus for both of them, Molly is now so impressed by her daughter's ability to ask for a variety of healthy foods that there is no longer any fighting between them.

Edith was a mom who raised her hand during the question period following a seminar I gave. She stated that her daughter, Toni, was a very intelligent nine-year-old whose maturity had earned her a certain degree of independence and respect from her parents. For the most part, Toni was a great eater, but she absolutely refused to eat any dairy. On this issue, she was unrelenting, refusing even to try any other calcium-rich food options. Her parents were really beginning to worry, and so I proposed that Edith present the situation to Toni pretty much as it was and consider setting some limits in the following way:

1. Despite Toni's maturity, she was not behaving maturely by refusing to find any options for calcium. In fact, she was taking poor care of her body and depriving it of something it absolutely needed.

2. If she was unable to make any choices that would help her to take better care of her body, she would lose some

of the privileges that she earned by being responsible. Her parents could not reward her for the independence and maturity she was showing in other areas when she was behaving so carelessly toward her own body and not taking care of it.

The basic communication was: "It is your job to take good care of your body, but if you cannot do that, then we as your parents are going to move in and present some limits." They had to be the bad guys. And, lo and behold, when they presented the situation that way, Toni found some calcium-rich foods she was willing to eat and thereby kept the privileges she'd earned.

Our kids need to learn how to make their own decisions, but we as parents need to know when to say no. By doing that, we save them from feeling overwhelmed with the enormity of making decisions whose consequences are beyond their comprehension. For example, Toni couldn't possibly connect to the fact that her bones wouldn't grow well if she didn't have adequate calcium, but she certainly could connect to the fact that if she continued to behave irresponsibly toward her body, her parents were going to move in and set limits to make sure she did what was necessary.

Setting Limits Means Being Willing to Be the Bad Guy

We need to set limits in order for our children to begin having any understanding of the consequences of their actions and, most important, to become familiar with the idea and feeling of disappointment when they do not get what they want. I laugh when I think of one of my mentors, who joked, "It's all downhill after three months!"—meaning that for the first three months of an infant's life, we give him exactly what he needs: we feed him when he cries for food, we hold him and rock him to sleep, we try to tune in and give him exactly what he wants. But then suddenly reality sets in, and we realize we have to begin establishing some rules and parameters. When we try to sleep train our baby and/or establish some sort of feeding schedule, we are confronted for the first time with what it feels like to be the bad guy. We know instinctively that we need to establish certain limits so that our child will learn to sleep through the night or eat in a more regular way—but it's not always easy to follow through.

Children need to be disappointed by us. Young children think in black and white. When you say no, and they vehemently state "I hate you!" they are simply declaring how they feel in that moment. As they mature, they are better able to integrate the two emotional states: their feelings of disappointment at not getting what they want (the bad feelings) and their satisfaction at receiving what they want (the good feelings), which are often tied to feeling loved by you. They become able to manage their intense negative feelings, which further enables them to accept the limits you set and, most important, stay connected to your loving them. Doing those two things helps them learn how to soothe themselves in the face of strong emotions.

Another reason it is so important to say no and sometimes disappoint our children is that having limits helps them feel safe. When children have too much power and know they can manipulate their parents through acting out, they end up feeling very unsafe. Kids are far from dumb; they know they shouldn't be in charge! As parents, you need to feel confident about setting limits that keep your children safe in order for them to practice their decision making.

Recently, I was working with John and Maryanne, a couple who were having some difficulties setting limits around various issues with their youngest child, Mason, who was a Food Demander. John felt strongly that Maryanne was being too permissive and that they should set up more structure because their son's demands were disturbing the family's mealtime. Maryanne, however, was struggling with the idea of setting limits with her six-year-old because she hated to see him disappointed and didn't want to be the bad guy. John resented Maryanne's reluctance to stick to their parameters and believed that her refusal to cooperate was exacerbating the situation with Mason.

With some encouragement from me, Maryanne and John began to work together to set limits. One of their rules was to allow all their children one treat a day. A few days later, Maryanne told me what had happened when she struggled to help Mason make a decision and learn from its outcome. When she had picked him up from school, the ice cream truck was outside. He begged her for an ice cream, and she wanted to say yes, but she knew they were having cake that night to celebrate John's birthday, and she remembered how much they had struggled to establish the one-treat-a-day rule, so she didn't want to relent. When she said no, Mason begged and whined until finally she decided she would say yes, but that she would also guide him to figure out which choice he wanted by telling him that he wouldn't be able to have cake that evening if he had ice cream now. Which would he prefer? He chose the ice cream.

Sure enough, that evening Mason begged for a piece of cake. It practically killed her, but Maryanne said no, reminding him of the choice he had made earlier that day. She found that by simply holding on to the knowledge that this was the decision her son had made, she was also able to set limits despite his whining and to encourage him to take responsibility for his choice. She also pointed out to Mason that in the future he might think back on this time and make a different choice. Sure enough, Maryanne was able to use the cake episode as a reminder when the ice cream truck came around again, and Mason felt more confident in making the choices he had: ice cream now or dessert later.

What is most important here is that John and Maryanne figured out a way to negotiate their differences, set the parameters with which they were both comfortable, and give their child some freedom to make his own decisions. In time, a lot of the fighting was defused, and the couple got along better, too. Being the bad guy was not easy at first, but with experience both Maryanne and Mason became more comfortable with the family parameters, and Maryanne felt less like the bad guy as she saw the positive results of shifting some of the responsibility to her son.

Letting Children Make Decisions—Including Ones You May Think Are Bad

It's important for parents to let their children make their own decisions, even bad ones, which is why it's so important to make sure you also set parameters that will keep them safe. But watching or even anticipating our children making a mistake and feeling bad about it can be anything from frustrating to excruciating. It's our natural instinct to want to swoop down and "rescue" our children from the consequences of their mistakes or bad decisions. As most of us know by now, however, such rescuing often results in children's never learning how to pick themselves up and move on from mistakes or disappointments. What they will learn, instead, is to distrust themselves, and as a result, they are more likely to get stuck feeling ashamed or disappointed. In addition to which you will be communicating to them that you don't think they can handle states of sadness, disappointment, and anxiety. You will be telling them that these are very dangerous states of mind and therefore to be avoided at all costs, which of course is impossible. For all these reasons, parents who rescue kids are actually doing them a disservice rather than a service.

If, on the other hand, you can let go of some of your control by giving your child the opportunity to make a choice, you are giving the gift of helping them develop judgment and decision-making skills, which is an ego strengthener that will bolster her self-esteem and self-confidence—two key building blocks that prevent a lifetime of eating problems.

Here are some questions to use as guidelines for helping your kids be responsible for their choices, even those you may think of as bad:

1. Is this a situation that will put my child in physical danger?
2. What will be the consequences for me, if I give my child these choices?
3. Can I as a parent live with whatever choice my child may make?
4. Can I truly support my child's decision and maintain a nonjudgmental attitude, simply helping her observe the outcome of her choice?
5. Can I as a parent remain firm in my limit setting in the face of the possibility that my child may whine, have a tantrum, or display some other emotional reaction?
6. Can I remember to reinforce the lesson with a light touch instead of reminding her of her mistake in a "told you so" way?
7. Can I remember to use this as an opportunity for her to learn from her decision?
8. Can I remember to teach my child that very few decisions create terrible mistakes?

Helping Kids Decide What They Are Hungry For

We all have days when we want something chewy or something sweet. Other days we want something salty or crunchy. Some meals we feel like having salad; other meals, we just need to have that steak. How do we make these decisions about what to eat? Most young children still have a

Don't Eat Around the Bush

YOU KNOW THOSE DAYS when just one particular food will satisfy you? Perhaps a Snickers bar or a bowl of ice cream or potato chips? You know you are feeling anxious, blue, whatever, and that you may even be eating emotionally, but you also know it's only that particular food that will satisfy. I urge my clients to predict what will happen if they do not give themselves that food. Certainly on some days you can make a different choice and the craving will go away. But on others, you may start out eating an apple, then carrots, then a bowl of cereal, then almonds, and so on—all in an effort to satisfy that craving! And then finally, at the end of it all, you eat the Snickers bar anyway. Well, kids are the same and have cravings as well. What you want to teach them is balance and sound nutrition. But it is also important to teach them to listen to what they need and not deprive themselves. Remember the studies mentioned in chapter one about how restricting backfires.

natural, built-in sense of what their bodies need. But as we saw in chapter five, this connection to their bodies can become dulled. Nevertheless, I have seen again and again in my practice that when they are given access to a range of foods in all categories—vegetables, starches, meat, fish, fruit, sweets—children will eventually begin to reconnect with their bodies and eat both moderately and nutritiously. They may, however, need your help figuring out what they want to eat. Of course they always tell us what they don't want, right? No, no, and no!

The Ouija Game is an easy exercise that will help you

guide your children to figure out exactly what they want to eat. It will help children zero in on what their tummies feel like, what food they are in the mood for, and so on. In the same way that we pass our hands over a Ouija board in hopes of discovering some kind of hidden truth to our lives, this exercise teaches children to "pass their minds over their bodies" to determine its needs and desires. Based on the idea that the body does know what food it needs, the Ouija Game is a fun way to help your child get in touch with his appetite, which in turn will strengthen his belly-head connection.

You probably use this technique daily without even realizing it. Have you ever sat in a restaurant with a menu in front of you, trying to determine what to choose from the list of options? You scan your eyes down the menu, imagining each dish in your mouth, then going down your throat into your stomach. If your body is craving meat and mashed potatoes (something heavy, in other words), that dish will immediately appeal to you when you visualize it. If, however, your body needs crunchy vegetables with fiber, a salad may be more appealing. This cluing in to your "food mood" is exactly what you can teach your children with the Ouija Game.

The Ouija Game Exercise

Try asking your child such questions as:

- "Do you feel like having something hot or cold? Mushy or crispy? Light or heavy?"
- "Let's think of the foods you've been eating recently to see what your body might need." Then go through the possibilities together.

Try to get your child to remember the food-body connection by asking questions such as:

- "Do you think your body has gotten what it needs to keep its muscles strong so you can really go for it at that soccer game this afternoon?"
- "What about your bones? I know you want to grow into that skirt Grandma sent you. Has your body gotten enough calcium to help your bones grow? Let's think of some foods that will help it do that: yogurt, broccoli, strawberries, milk, cheese, beans."

If you sense that your child's energy tends to flag an hour or so after eating, perhaps her meals or snacks are too carb-heavy and she needs more protein. (Remember that too many carbs can cause blood sugar to spike and then drop.)

- Remind her of this connection and then offer some ideas for protein, such as nuts, a peanut butter and jelly sandwich, cheese, or even a hot dog if she likes them!

The key to this exercise is to help your children get involved in making their own decisions about which foods help their bodies grow in different ways. By reinforcing the nutritional information you've given them and encouraging your children to take charge of all or part of the decision-making process, they will begin to "own" their bodies in a whole new way. And once they know that it is their job to feed their bodies, they will also realize they are the expert on what their bodies need.

Reinforcing Nutrition Lessons

THROUGHOUT ALL THE STEPS you take to teach your kids how to eat for life, you need to continue to integrate and reinforce information about nutrition. This is the foundation upon which they will build all their knowledge about how to take care of their own bodies. Here are some suggestions for helping children make the connection between what they eat and how best to take care of their bodies:

1. Find the particular activity your child loves best.

2. If he needs bone growth, teach him about those foods that give him calcium to help his bones to grow, really making the connection between those foods and the desired activity.

3. If he continues to demand certain foods, remind him that while the food he's asking for is fun to eat, it's not going to do much to help him grow taller or have the muscle strength to climb a tree (again, tailor your example to the specific activity you know your child loves best).

4. Give him room to choose within the foods that help develop muscle strength, bone strength, and so on.

5. Remind him that of course he can have a treat that day, but that he also needs to give his body the fuel it requires to do what he wants it to do.

6. If your child is very young, you will need to offer him choices. For example, you can offer him yogurt or cheese or pasta or chicken fingers—pick something you know he likes and that has some nutritional value, and limit the choices to perhaps three items.

7. If the child still refuses to eat or choose, state that he must not be hungry. Then reinforce that he must be listening to his body, and when he becomes hungry he might have a better idea of what he wants because the signal from his body will be louder.

8. If your child continues to ask for dessert, ask him to do a body check, prompting him with such questions as, "How hungry are you? Where is the hunger? In your stomach?" If he discovers that he is still hungry, suggest that he fill up by eating more of his meal, after which he can have dessert.

It Takes Practice

Children don't learn the four steps to eating for life overnight. They need practice, encouragement, and a lot of reinforcement from their parents. Rayna was a nine-year-old girl at the time I met her and her family. Her parents were frustrated and worried because Rayna had been progressively gaining weight since the age of seven. Although she had always been slightly chubby, her weight gain had accelerated over the previous two years. Her parents also noticed that Rayna was becoming increasingly unhappy with herself, frequently making critical comments about her body and saying that she wanted to lose weight. They had consulted an endocrinologist and then a nutritionist. And while Rayna had initially lost weight by following the plan the nutritionist provided, she lost her motivation after several weeks and began to regain the weight. That's when the nutritionist referred Rayna to me.

When the family and I met, we discovered that every time Rayna felt deprived because she wanted to be eating the same foods as her friends (Chinese food, french fries, and so on), she would go to the fridge when she knew her parents weren't looking and secretly eat the foods she knew she "shouldn't" have. Rayna admitted to me that on these occasions, she was trying desperately to feed herself as much as she could because she truly believed that the next day she would "be good, and absolutely not touch those foods again." As a result, she barely ever tasted what she was eating.

As we worked together, it became clear that "being good tomorrow" was interfering with Rayna's ability to stop eating those foods when she was full. (In fact she barely even noticed whether she was hungry or full, and we joked that she was eating on autopilot!) Additionally and equally important, Rayna began to describe the feelings she had when she craved a "bad food" and "gave in." (Can you hear the rigid standards she set for herself?) She said she felt disappointed in herself, ashamed, and also that she knew that her parents were feeling terribly disappointed in her. In fact she could hardly bear to look at their faces as she described this to me. We were able to conclude the following:

1. When she felt ashamed, she tried to fix it by thinking immediately: "I'll be good tomorrow; I will definitely lose this weight!"
2. She would then spend several minutes feeling terrible about herself and revert to thinking, "I am a failure," quickly losing any motivation to change her behavior.

3. The consequence was that she would again turn to food to soothe her feelings of shame and discomfort, and the negative cycle would continue.

The first way we decided to help Rayna was by guiding her to reconnect with her body's signals of fullness and hunger. She needed to reset her satiety signal to perfectly comfortable (number 5) by knowing that she could have ACCESS to eating the foods she loved in moderation so that she no longer felt compelled to stuff them down because they would not be available tomorrow. She needed to learn how to distinguish among feelings of sadness, feelings of failure, and feelings of hunger, and she needed to learn to FEEL her feelings, so that she would not soothe her emotions with food.

Given that Rayna was feeling deprived when she was with her friends who were eating fries and Chinese food, I worked with her to expand the repertoire of foods she could eat. The key for Rayna was to learn how to stop overeating these so-called bad foods. I also worked with her parents to allow Rayna access to the foods if she wanted, encouraging them to help her assume responsibility for stopping when she was full.

I then showed Rayna the Hunger-Fullness scale. Her instructions were that she needed to take responsibility for listening to the signals within her body. She used the Waiting Game and kept checking in with her body, knowing that she could always eat more of the food she loved the next day.

As much as Rayna understood and paid attention to her signals, however, she was still having trouble managing the decisions. She needed to learn how to deal with the intense emotions she would have at times: feelings of disappointment if she didn't do as well as she had thought she should (with eating, with school, with friends). To do that, she learned to identify her feelings and used the Wave Exercise to increase her ability to WAIT through them, which helped decrease her use of food to soothe herself. But she also had to figure out other ways to feel better when she was having a tough time. I suggested that Rayna do the following Balance Sheet Exercise, to help her think a bit more about the different choices she could make whenever she began to notice the feelings that usually triggered her eating.

Balance Sheet Exercise

On one side of the Balance Sheet, she listed the positive and negative consequences of eating when she felt terrible:

- Positive: immediate halt to those thoughts and feelings.
- Negative: ongoing weight gain and reinforcement of negative feelings about herself.

On the other side of the balance sheet, I instructed her to write down the positives and negatives of *not* eating when feeling terrible:

- Positive: a feeling of competence and the development of a new skill, one that would help her comfort herself.
- Positive: ultimately taking in fewer calories and, therefore, losing weight (her stated goal).

- Negative: the belief that feelings of anxiety and panic would last forever.

That last part, worrying that the feelings would last forever, is not to be underestimated and is probably why it's so difficult to change one's eating behavior and learn how to avoid using food for comfort. In fact, all the experts in the field of eating know that both restricting food and compulsively eating does reduce anxiety in the moment. The problem is that these are short-term solutions that produce long-term problems. You end up in a vicious cycle. The eating calms the anxiety but produces longer-term problems, such as weight gain, low self-esteem, decreased confidence in being able to wait, and a lack of skills to cope with feelings. Although it can be difficult to help kids sit with their anxiety, they do need to build skills and develop ways to manage their negative feelings in order to prevent them from using food to soothe themselves.

It was very important for both Rayna and her parents to understand that she was learning a new and very difficult skill. Like any learning process, this one would involve some effort, and certainly there would be times when it didn't work. The important thing is to know that it takes practice. I always tell clients that it is like building a new muscle. You can't expect it to be easy, but the muscle will get stronger with practice. You need to be realistic. The more pressure we took off Rayna, the more she took pressure off herself. She was then able to continue trying, even in the face of failure. By doing that, she eventually developed a new way of coping with her feelings, and in time relied less on food.

As Rayna's parents began to see that she was learning how to try, they were able to give her the support she needed without attempting to fix the problem for her. Rayna's parents learned to offer her room to feel disappointment without trying to rescue her. They began to have more confidence in her, and with the confidence she felt from them, she was able to begin making decisions for herself.

One of the feelings Rayna's mother was able to identify

Your Role in Creating a Confident Decision Maker

TO HELP GUIDE YOUR CHILDREN to become confident decision makers, try to

- be patient;
- validate their feelings;
- help them give names to their feelings—especially young children;
- know that understanding your child's feelings is not the same as being permissive;
- provide appropriate ways for your child to express his feelings;
- set limits and make sure your child understands the consequences of her actions;
- follow through on the limits you set—you can empathize with your child's frustration, but do not change the consequences.

in herself was how pained she felt when Rayna became upset. She couldn't bear to see Rayna feeling so bad about herself. I helped her understand both that it is unavoidable at times for our children to feel bad about themselves, and that Rayna could learn not to lose touch with those parts of herself she felt good about if she could decrease the behavior that was reinforcing the bad feeling to begin with.

Within about eight months, Rayna was able to achieve an appropriate body weight with which she felt comfortable. She remains connected to her body's signals and now has tools for dealing with the day-to-day stresses and emotions in her life. She has been able to maintain the weight loss and is on the growth curve she had been on until the age of seven. It has been three years now, and Rayna knows how to eat for life.

A Quick Review

Teaching our children how to become confident decision makers is all about balance. Our children need our guidance, and they sometimes need to be told what to do. But they also need our permission and encouragement to take risks, make choices, and live with consequences that may not be so great. So remember to try to be flexible.

You cannot always let your children make their own decisions. Pick the situations. Figure out how deleterious it is for them to do what they are doing, and help them think the situation through in a nonjudgmental way. At the same time, don't be afraid to let them know if you really think something is a bad idea. Even if you don't state it, you will be communicating this anyway, and they will feel your disapproval. This will impact their ability to accept the consequences of their decisions. And you will be sending them a double message: "I am letting you make the decision but I think it is not a very smart one."

You have to be very careful to establish parameters you can live with so that you don't wind up saying "I told you so." Your effort to give your children freedom and encouragement needs to be genuine. If it isn't, they will know it. They need to feel that you respect them and that as they learn to accept consequences and take more responsibility, you will be impressed by them!

Consider these important points as you begin to teach your children the skills they need to make confident decisions:

1. You are the parent.
2. You know more than your child and can predict the outcome of his decisions. Do not be afraid to guide your children.
3. Make sure a child's decision is safe. A young child cannot foresee the outcome of his choices in the same way as an older child. He needs to be directed with parameters and suggestions.
4. Your child needs you to be the bad guy at times in order for him to learn how to be mad at you. By accepting that role you help your child avoid feeling overwhelmed by issues he cannot make sense of, especially feelings of shame.
5. Be direct when you think your child might be considering making a poor decision. Otherwise you will be

sending him a double message, and he will feel your silent criticism while you are telling him that he can make his own decisions.

6. Remember that your children want your approval as they are figuring out their way through the world by making decisions. Do not be afraid to guide them.

PART THREE

Establishing Parameters That Work for You

CHAPTER EIGHT

Finding Your Comfort Zone

A S YOU BEGIN TO UNDERSTAND your own food legacy and teach your children the four steps to eating for life, you will naturally come to a place where you become more conscious of the parameters or rules you want to establish and reinforce in your household. Throughout the previous chapters, you have been figuring out which rules work for your children and which ones don't. You have been learning how to offer them some choices without giving them complete freedom, which is one of the tightropes we all walk as parents.

Now you will have an opportunity to review not only where your kids are in terms of their eating behavior but also where you are as the parent in charge of establishing clear rules and parameters. Perhaps you have already decided on the food rules in your house; perhaps you find yourself vacillating between being rigid and being flexible; or perhaps you feel that you are up a stream without a paddle. In this chapter, I will help you to clarify the rules and parameters that work for you and to create a family food style that fits.

Keeping Your Child in Perspective

Review your child's developmental stage and eating style so that you can be objective about her needs and behavior around food. Here are a few questions to consider:

1. Are you still worried about your child's health? Determine if she is healthy and on her growth curve. If you still have questions, consult your physician.

2. Are you comfortable with your child's body type? If you are uncomfortable because your daughter is large for a girl or your son small for a boy, try to acknowledge your feelings of discomfort. If you don't acknowledge your own discomfort, you may unwittingly contribute to your child's over- or undereating. Be aware of whether you are trying to overcontrol your child's eating. If you need help learning how to refrain from making critical comments, seek professional support to sort through your own feelings. It will help your child immensely.

3. Whose problem is it? Is your child's eating behavior developmentally appropriate? In keeping with his eating style? Is this eating style different from your own? Try to separate your feelings from your child's eating behavior in order to establish whether he is indeed developing any habits that might be interfering with his ability to eat for life.

4. Are your children able to self-regulate or do they have trouble stopping when they are full? Do you have to pull the plate away in order for them to stop eating?

Review Step Two to help your children reboot the connection between the belly and the head.

5. If your child is a picky eater or doesn't eat a lot, think about your own or your partner's eating habits when you were children. Were either of you picky eaters? Were or are you both small in stature? Make sure you are being objective and setting up realistic standards for your child to follow.

6. Has your child begun to make her own food choices? Has she begun to assume responsibility for her own body?

7. Does your child follow your rules and guidelines without question? Do you think this compliance means she wants to please you or does it mean that she has absorbed the nutritional information you've been giving her? If you think your child may be too compliant, begin to reinforce her ability to make her own choices about food by giving her options for what and when to eat or the choice to plan some meals.

8. If your children continue to balk at your rules and fight you on the parameters you have established, are they being temperamentally strong-willed, caught up in their desire to challenge you, or are they exercising their wish to make some of their own food choices? If you think they may be trying to challenge you, you can introduce and reinforce more choices in order to defuse their motivation to fight.

9. Is your child able to create even more battles over meals or snacks because you and your partner have set conflicting rules? If so, try to compromise so that the two of you can present a more united front.

Establishing Your Rules

PARENTS TEND TO MAKE rules with regard to several general areas:

- Eating with the television on
- Reading at the table
- Sitting at the table together as a family
- Eating together
- Eating three meals a day
- Snacks, sugar, and junk food
- Table manners
- Leaving the table

It's not always easy to clarify our feelings about our children's eating behavior. But the more often you return to these points of reference, the more likely it is that you will remain objective about what is going on with your kids at any given time. And remember, kids change all the time!

Questions to Help You Consider Your Rules and Parameters

Although more than likely you have already made many of these decisions, it may be helpful to review the following questions as a way to clarify how you feel about the various aspects of dealing with food and kids. Your rules will probably evolve and adapt as your children develop; re-member that the older they get, the more civilized they be-come. And be realistic. It may not be worth your effort to set up rules for a one-and-a-half-year-old who cannot sit still for more than the five minutes it takes for her to eat. Although young children can learn to sit longer in time, you don't want to set yourself up to be frustrated.

You can also try out various rules before deciding on any one set of parameters. You can always change your mind. Pick the nonnegotiables that are in keeping with your own value system, concerns, and general guidelines, and leave yourself room for flexibility. If you, your partner, and your children are clear about the nonnegotiables, you will feel more comfortable being flexible about the guidelines you establish. For example, are you able to set a definite rule about the time the kitchen closes so that your child does not manipulate you with frantic cries of "But I am hungry now!" just before bedtime? How comfortable do you feel stating in response, "You had your chance to eat at dinnertime; if you are hungry when you go to bed, you will eat more tomor-row, and maybe next time you will eat more when the kitchen is still open"? Are you being held hostage to the kitchen because you are worried that your child will go to bed hungry? Do you still think that all meals need to be com-pletely nutritious? While some parents may have the time to cook all the family meals, offering their children a range of wholesome, organic foods every night, they are not in the majority. Most parents have neither the time nor the energy to pull off such a coup. And there are plenty of parents whose children are perfectly healthy in spite of eating meals that consist of pizza, hot dogs, and macaroni and cheese.

You need to be flexible with the rules you set so that you don't drive yourself completely crazy. You may have a long list of nonnegotiables, or you may feel more comfortable staying flexible. The point is to figure out what you are comfortable with and what works best for your children. Remember, consistent parenting is never 100 percent. If you stray from your parameters occasionally—either on a whim or for a special occasion—your children will not suddenly forget the rules. Consider the following questions as you review the parameters you wish to establish with your children:

1. How permissive or restrictive do you want to be?
2. Have you figured out what food rules you want to establish in your household? Are your kids clear about how often they can have dessert? Do you want your kids to try at least one bite of something new before deciding they don't like a particular food? How many choices do you want to offer if your children are not interested in the meal you have prepared?
3. Have you begun to talk regularly about nutrition with your kids, using the Food Pyramid as a guide and reference?
4. Are you comfortable with your children's intake of nutritious foods on a biweekly basis?
5. Are you comfortable with the amount of sugar and other sweet foods they eat?
6. How important is it to you that meals be served at regularly scheduled times?
7. How comfortable are you with a child who likes to graze as opposed to eating three square meals a day?

8. Are you comfortable establishing some rules as basic guidelines and loosening up on weekends or special occasions? Is your partner comfortable with this as well? Have you clarified to your children your ability to be flexible on special occasions?

9. Are you comfortable mixing up the order of the meals? For example, do you allow your children to have pizza and ice cream for breakfast if they wish, with the understanding they won't be able to have dessert after dinner?

10. Are you encouraging your children to help establish healthy eating habits and give you ideas for what they would like to eat? Do they help you shop for groceries? Do they help you cook?

11. Do you have rules about your children's needing to finish all the food on their plate? How comfortable are you letting them pick their own portion sizes and allowing them to figure out how much food their bodies might be wanting, even if that amount varies?

12. Are you modeling the idea of "eating when you are hungry, stopping when you are full"? Are you reinforcing the idea that sometimes their head may want more when their belly has already had enough?

There Is No Such Thing as Perfection

NO MATTER HOW clear you are or how flexible or strict, there will be days when your children are simply offtrack when it comes to eating and food.

Are You Ready to Let Go?

Throughout this process, I have been encouraging you to help your children become confident decision makers by giving them some responsibility for making their own food choices. Parents who are uncomfortable with letting go of control are usually those who are also most rigid about the rules they set. Although as the parent you need to make such rules, and you have to be comfortable with them, you also need to know when to allow for flexibility and freedom so your children can make some of their own decisions about food.

If you want your children to eat well for life and not obsess about food, it is important to model a certain freedom with food—even if you have to fake it at times. This means trying very hard to stay away from comments about good or bad foods, and trying to separate your own issues

Consider Shelving the Rules on Weekends

I BELIEVE STRONGLY in downtime on weekends. In our house, this is when we loosen up on any rules we have during the week, such as not eating in front of the television and sitting down together at the table. On weekends, I allow my children to eat in front of the television and to change the general order of meals—pizza for breakfast, cereal for dinner, and so on. We all need to relax at times and have a change of pace.

or worries about weight gain, nutrition intake, and other concerns from the way you deal with your children's eating issues. If you truly enjoy food and want your children to share that enjoyment, then continue to model your enthusiasm about food, encourage your children to develop their own tastes, and respect their appetite, knowing that eventually your values will more than likely take hold.

Sometimes, however, you will have to reassess whether what you are doing is working. One mother shared with me that the rule in her house had always been that everyone had to try one bite of a new food before deciding she didn't like it. While she understood the logic of the rule she had grown up with, she had always found that it in fact made her more resistant to really being open to new foods, and therefore she decided not to impose this rule on her children. She discovered that by backing off, her kids ended up being very curious about different foods.

Another mother, Sue, let me know that her mother had been exceptionally rigid about the food in their house, but that they were allowed to have junk food and sugar outside the house. While Sue had felt that this same rule would work with her three children, she found that her very active, picky four-year-old became too demanding of sweet foods once she had access to them at playgroups. Sue and her husband, Jim, who is also rigid about his own diet, then had to figure out how to adapt their rules so that they worked for the entire family. They wanted to model healthy eating, but they didn't want to create a sugar baby by being too rigid. They decided to allow sugar and sweets in the house with the rule that the children could have dessert three times per week, and within two weeks, their daughter began to back off demanding sugar.

This situation brought Sue face-to-face with her family food legacy. What she discovered when she thought through the situation was that although she felt good about her mother's parenting style, she realized that she had not taken into account the developmental stage of her four-year-old daughter. Before becoming more flexible, Sue had to face her own feelings about not being a "good" mother. By working through the steps, and gaining more confidence in her daughter's ability to adapt to certain rules within a framework that allowed choice and freedom, Sue learned that part of being a good parent is being responsive and flexible to the changing needs of your children. Ultimately, she and Jim were able to arrive at a set of values they wanted to establish for their family without turning each meal into a battle.

If you are still having trouble letting go of your worry, it is possible that your concerns stem not from your children's situation but from your own food legacy and the food issues with which you continue to struggle. In my clinical experience working with all sorts of families, this is probably the area where most adults have the greatest difficulty. It is crucial that you get to know your own food legacy so that you can take the necessary steps to separate your own food issues from your children's eating behavior (as described in chapter one). Until you do that, your worries may continue unnecessarily and unabated. However, you may need additional assistance. If this is the case, I recommend that you seek out a professional or therapist who can guide you as you untangle this often confusing web.

Partner Differences

Much of the frustration and headache of feeding our children stems from partners' having different approaches. In my practice, I have found it rare to see both parents thinking exactly alike when it comes to food. For instance, one may be ready to give her daughter five lollipops if she asks for them while the other may feel that even one lollipop is excessive. One parent may feel strongly that dessert before dinner or lunch is a no-no, while the other may feel that it's not the end of the world. The parents who have the most success navigating such stark differences in attitude toward sugar and other controversial foods are those who keep in mind that their primary goal is to help their children learn to eat for life.

Both parents need to realize how quickly kids can gravitate to making food a power issue (remember that they're masters at detecting your agendas!) and avoid unwittingly setting up a struggle between themselves. Remember, we all feel fiercely protective of our parenting beliefs and therefore can easily become vulnerable to threats in this domain.

An anecdote from my practice may help you to manage such partner differences. Connie, the mother of five-year-old Sarah, came to me complaining that her daughter had recently been exposed to more sweets when she started attending birthday parties. A clear reaction to this new, more intense exposure to sweets was that Sarah was suddenly wanting more snacks of this kind, and sometimes she was even asking for them before dinner.

Connie herself had struggled with an eating disorder as

a teenager and young adult and found that when she was less restrictive about what she let herself eat, she became much less preoccupied with food and much happier about eating in general. As a result, she had always tried to be less restrictive with her children to avoid triggering disordered eating in them.

Her husband, Karl, however, was raised by parents who served only health food, restricting most sweets. As a result, he had very strong negative ideas about sugar and believed that dessert came only *after* a meal, if at all.

When I began asking Connie how Sarah interacted with her and her husband, she said something not too surprising. "Actually," Connie explained, "Sarah seems to be more demanding of cookies or candy with Karl and less demanding with me." I asked her to describe her own behavior with her daughter, and it appeared to be somewhat flexible. Connie believed that Sarah would naturally self-regulate if she were allowed to do so. But when she explained this approach to her husband, he was completely against it.

Yet in the shared hope of helping their daughter, Karl agreed to compromise so that they could function as a team. And when Sarah started taking care of her body by selecting good fuel, Karl began to see that she did not, in fact, "spoil her appetite" by having a cookie first. Gradually he felt more confident about being a bit more flexible, particularly when Connie pointed out that Sarah became even more demanding about sugar when she was with him. Sensing his discomfort and rigidity about sugar, she would try to "push his buttons"—and usually win! Once both her parents were "on the same page," Sarah was also better able to understand the rules, and in time she created less of a fight.

Sometimes, however, there is one parent who is adamantly opposed to the idea of his or her children having any control or decision-making power with regard to food. Such was the case in another family with whom I worked. Casey and Mark came to see me because they were very worried about their three-year-old son, Jack, who was driving them crazy with his demands for candy and cookies. Casey was much more comfortable giving Jack cookies when he asked for them, knowing that eventually he would eat other, more nutritious food. But Mark would become infuriated with his son. When I asked Mark about what was making him so angry, he said, "Jack is being disrespectful. If I ever acted that way to my parents, I would have been hammered." Mark's anger was being triggered not only by Jack's behavior but also by Casey's flexibility. In his mind, Casey was "just giving in" to Jack.

Before this couple was able to establish a middle ground between the wife's flexibility and the husband's rigidity, Mark had to do a little work. He needed to look at why he had been reacting so strongly to his son's behavior. Once Mark was able to see that Jack wasn't *intending* to be disrespectful, but was merely acting like any demanding three-and-a-half-year-old, he was able to calm down. And he also came to realize that he was actually feeling resentful of his son's freedom, given all the restrictions he experienced as a child. When he learned to recognize Jack's desire for separation and individuation, Mark found he could hold on to his no without losing his cool.

We are often drawn to our partners because they are

different from and complement us. And it is frequently those very qualities we fell in love with that also drive us crazy during stressful parenting times. We find ourselves saying, "I cannot believe she doesn't see it my way!" "I can't believe he doesn't even hear their screaming!" "He is so laid-back that I am always having to be the bad guy!"

If this is the case in your household, it is important to recognize and address your differences and the tensions they create. Children, of course, will go to the parent who doesn't say no, which will cause fights and undermine any parameters that have been set. Our kids need us to work as a team because it helps them feel safe. You must, therefore, come up with a bit of a middle ground, even if your styles are different. Find parameters that are comfortable for you both, and remember, these rules don't have to be too rigid. Finding a middle ground does not mean you have to believe in the exact same thing; and you don't always have to do the exact same thing. But the more children are able to see their parents working as a team, the less tension there will be and the less able they will be to set up power struggles.

If parents are able to keep their primary goal in mind (teaching their kids to eat for life), they can be more effective at negotiating differences between themselves and establishing parameters that are mutually acceptable. As you and your partner begin this process of teaching your kids to eat for life, ask yourselves these questions:

1. What particular rules do you feel absolutely dogmatic about? Which of these does your partner agree with? If choosing either position is unrealistic, discuss how

you can support each other's point of view with the shared goal of teaching your kids how to eat for life. One way to reach a compromise in the area of food is to turn to other areas—bedtime, evening time, one person's resentment at always being the disciplinarian (or bad guy). Partners have a lot of areas in which they can focus their energy and find creative solutions, leaving more room to compromise in the area of food.

2. What are the differences between you, and how are you going to reconcile them so that you can provide one set of expectations for your children? Again, it is about give-and-take; fair does not mean exactly equal all the time. Your child needs you to work as a team.

3. Is there room for differences between you?

4. Is there something about your family food legacy or your own food attitudes that is causing you to be so rigid? Often when partners respond strongly to each other's differing attitudes or points of view, they are actually reacting to their own food issues. By taking a closer look at your own background (or that of your partner), you might be able to defuse some of the tension created by your markedly different approaches to food.

Dealing with Intrusive Grandparents and Other Opinionated Adults

As parents, we are forced to get used to our children's being influenced by other people, especially other adults. And sometimes even the best-meaning of these adults can challenge our patience. Indeed, when we are confronted by a grandparent, caregiver, teacher, or babysitter who is critical of our rules or gives contradictory advice to our children, how are we supposed to respond? As I mentioned earlier, the clearer and surer you are of your own parameters, the more you can insist on your point of view without wavering. But even the most tenacious of us may wilt under a little pressure.

From speaking with hundreds of parents, I've determined that grandparents are the most difficult to deal with. They know us best, tend to get under our skin most easily and quickly, and often have the ability to make us feel like teenagers all over again! Trust your own parenting style and know that you have the most influence on your child's eating behavior. Here are some tips:

1. Explain to your parents that you are very clear and comfortable with the process of teaching your kids how to eat for life.
2. Offer to share this book with them so they become more familiar with the reasons behind some of your actions and parameters.
3. Remind them of how they dealt with your food issues and that their strategies didn't necessarily work.
4. Remind them that your kids are yours, not theirs.
5. If your children's grandparents are more permissive than you, try to give your children room when in their care. And remember, if your children know the rules of your household, they will not forget them just because they spend a weekend or even two weeks with their grandparents!

6. If you are less than comfortable dealing with your in-laws, have your partner talk directly with his or her parents about the parameters around eating in your household.

How to Work with Your Current Babysitter

Babysitters, nannies, and caregivers can also present challenges to our peace of mind as we teach our kids how to eat for life. I have worked with roughly five babysitters since the birth of my first daughter. All of them (with the exception of one nightmare) were terrific in different ways. Yet I've had to give each one a bit of coaching to help her understand how I wanted her to deal with my kids and food. If you would like your babysitter or other caregivers to follow your approach to feeding your children, here are some areas you may want to discuss with them:

1. Discuss the fact that you are trying to help your children develop a healthy relationship with food and strengthen their ability to make decisions about their food choices.
2. Find out if she has been using treats as rewards. Let her know that, of course, she will do this from time to time and that you will not be upset if she withholds an ice cream because your child is misbehaving. But tell her that, in general, you want to avoid using desserts as rewards or punishment. Discuss other strategies she can use instead.
3. Find out if she has been trying to get your child to eat his vegetables with the one-more-bite routine. Explain that you are trying to encourage your child to be moti-

vated to take good care of himself and to make good choices about nutrition. Refer to chapter four on nutrition to give her guidelines on how to talk with your child. Encourage her to let the child figure out how much to eat, reinforcing his ability to take good care of his body. And remind the caregiver not to fall back on the "if you take one more bite of dinner, you can have dessert" strategy, which can undermine your goal of teaching your child how to think of all foods as good.

4. Share some of the dialogue that has worked for you, so the caregiver has specific guidelines to follow. This will also help her understand your general attitude and approach to working with your child.

5. Show the caregiver some of the exercises, in particular the Waiting Game (see page 132), to use with your children.

6. Explain how she can use the Food Pyramid (page 88) and the Hunger-Fullness scale (page 124) as references. Show her how your child is using them, and/or ask your child to show her. That way, you can see exactly how much (or little) your child is actually understanding about nutrition and the other steps to eating for life.

How to Interview Potential Caregivers

Whether you are in the process of hiring a caregiver or want to review your caregiver's plans for managing food with your children, it's important to be very clear about your expectations. Make sure in your interviews with potential caregivers that you get an idea of how they are used to feeding children. You want to be sure that if your ideas are very different from theirs, there is room for discussion and compromise. You can ask some of the following questions:

1. In the other jobs you have had, what were some of the guidelines or rules about eating for the children? Did you agree with these or disagree? If you were not comfortable, how did you handle it?
2. What are your ideas about how Johnny should eat? Do you have any particular ideas about how snacks or meals should be given?
3. If her ideas seem different from yours, you can state: "I like to work with my kids a bit differently, and I am trying to strengthen their ability to make good food choices for themselves. For example, I don't reward the kids with dessert for eating their vegetables. How willing would you be to hear a bit more about how I do things and try to do them a bit differently?" (Rarely will a candidate say no directly, but you can sense her general reception to this request by how she reacts to you.)

With these questions, you will get a clearer idea of whether or not your potential babysitter has particularly strong feelings about how kids should be fed. Then you can figure out how much guidance you will want to give her. Parents differ—some give a lot of flexibility to their caregivers, while others feel strongly that caregivers should follow their recommendations to the letter. What is most important is that you be clear about your guidelines and that the caregiver seems willing to adhere to those guidelines.

Creating Your Own Family Style

Most mealtimes in my home are rather chaotic. I am still trying to get my children to sit still for more than the ten minutes it takes them to shovel their food down their throats—never mind convincing them to wait for my husband and me to finish our meals so that we can "talk" during the once, maybe twice a week we can actually sit down together for mealtime!

Should I be upset that three very active young girls are unable to enjoy a leisurely meal? Should I become stressed about their seeming inability to enjoy the ritual of sitting down with their parents at the end of the day? Should I insist that they sit, behave, and listen until they're spoken to? These questions occur to me often because I have been very conscious of wanting my kids to learn that meals are something we sit down to together and share. Doing that was a part of my childhood that I felt very strongly I wanted to replicate in my household.

Every family has its own meal style. There is no right or wrong way to conduct a meal. Perhaps you prefer to prepare dinner or lunch for your kids and serve them first on stools around the kitchen counter, so that you and your partner can then sit down for a more enjoyable "adult" meal. Perhaps you like to make one night out of the week a more formal dinner, at which you sit down together in the dining room as a family, while the rest of the week you are more flexible, feeding your kids more casually. Maybe you are a family that rarely if ever sits down together for a meal.

What I have found to be most important for making mealtimes happy, enjoyable occasions for both parents and children is to create a style that works for your particular family. The components that come into play here are your and your partner's values, backgrounds, comforts, and the rituals you would like to pass on to your children. Often if there is one parent who feels more strongly about a particular ritual, while the other is more flexible or does not particularly care one way or another, the parent with the stronger preference sets the pace.

I must admit, however, that I am biased. To me, mealtimes are opportunities for families to connect. I think it is important to help our children have the positive experience of coming together in a ritualized way to do something that happens over and over. Sharing a meal is an easy way to ensure that your kids begin to talk with you, and it gives you a chance to tune in to them. We have a ritual "Good Thing, Bad Thing" routine in which each person in the family shares one good thing and one bad thing that happened to him or her that day. My kids love this game; it helps them sit still longer, and open up and talk about themselves.

As you decide how you want to conduct meals in your household, keep in mind that you may again confront partner differences. On the surface, Sean and Terry, a couple I worked with, appeared to have similar backgrounds: they both grew up in the suburbs of New York City, were of the same ethnic and religious heritage, and very much shared the same value system. But when it came to mealtimes, they couldn't have been more different from each other. Sean hated to sit down for dinner and often grabbed a burger on his way home, even though he knew Terry had fixed a roast chicken dinner with baked potatoes and vegetables. Sean would then arrive home and not understand why Terry was so upset that he "was not hungry."

The tension between them became even more charged when Terry began to feel that Sean was undermining her efforts to teach their three boys table manners. As she explained to me, "I came from a family in which we sat down most nights of the week to dinner. We were taught good table manners, how to sit through a meal, how to listen to others and wait for everyone to finish before we were excused. My parents were strict, but I value the lessons they taught us." When I asked Sean to describe his family mealtimes, he said, "What family meals? My father and mother never ate with us. My mother always fed the two youngest first, and the four oldest later. I hated most foods and would only eat spaghetti or hamburgers."

It was clear that when it came to mealtimes Sean and Terry were from two different planets. Did Sean see the value in teaching their sons to have table manners and to sit down together as a family? "Yes, but I think Terry is too tough on them," he told me. When I asked Terry to respond, she admitted, "I think I'm tough because everyone is running around not listening to me." Finally they agreed that their kids should learn manners and that spending time as a family was good for everyone. Together, they decided to select at least two nights a week when they would sit down together as a family. Terry would give Sean advance notice, and he would make a conscious effort to support her.

Nowadays, one of the main obstacles to creating a family eating style is the sense that everyone is too busy to sit down and have a meal together. Whether this lack of time and energy is the result of both parents' working, the tendency for kids to be busy with activities right up until, and sometimes through, the traditional "dinnertime," or the fact that a single parent does not get home until late, I hear from more and more parents who are stressed about how to approach mealtimes with their kids. As you begin to think about the family style you have developed or want to create, try to take the stress out of mealtimes by putting the emphasis on sitting together rather than on the food itself.

By doing that, you can avoid triggering power struggles about eating and help your children begin to associate eating with positive times rather than with stress. If one or more of your children does not want to eat, you can still sit and talk together for the allotted time. Even small children eventually grow up and will be able to sit longer.

Use the official mealtime as an occasion to relax together. You will be amazed how well you can stay connected to your kids simply by establishing this ritual.

As you become more and more comfortable with the choices you make about how you deal with your kids and food, the more likely it is that you will feel confident about your ability to solve eating-related problems as they occur. In the next chapter, I have selected twenty of the questions I most commonly receive from parents. These questions and my responses will provide a crib sheet for dealing on the spot with age-related and eating-style issues.

CHAPTER NINE

Commonly Asked Questions and Answers

1. The Midnight Waker

Q: *I worked really hard to teach my nine-month-old child to sleep through the night. But since I introduced solid foods and began trying to establish mealtimes, I have found that she wakes up in the middle of the night, at which point I give her a bottle because I'm afraid she is hungry. Now my good little sleeper is no longer sleeping through the night!*

A: While it may be difficult, it is important for kids to know that nighttime is not for eating. Try to give the child a bottle right at bedtime. Or offer less food (especially snacks) during the afternoon so she will be hungrier at dinnertime. When you feed children at night, their bodies develop the habit of waking up, expecting to be fed. I assure you, they will not starve if they go to bed a bit hungrier one night—even if they do wake up. Do what you did to sleep train your child, and she will probably eat more the next day!

2. The Baby Who Loses Interest in Eating

Q: My fifteen-month-old used to eat quite a variety of foods and now eats hardly anything. I am worried he is not getting enough nutrition, especially since he is off formula.

A: You can be reassured that it is entirely normal for children to lose interest in eating as they begin to use their developing motor skills to explore the world. If your physician reassures you that your son is perfectly healthy and you are still worried, know that little children need very little food. Their caloric needs are much less than we think. The little fistfuls of Goldfish or one spoonful of peanut butter and cup of milk add up for small tummies. Also, remind yourself that a child's nutritional needs are met on a one- to two-week basis, so children do not have to eat balanced meals every day. (See chapter four for more assurance and information on nutritional requirements.)

3. The Grazer

Q: I'm concerned that my twenty-one-month-old is eating all day long. She doesn't stop eating snacks and then she barely eats at dinner. What should I do?

A: I've heard this from many parents of children that age. In part, you are probably concerned because you want to help your child move toward sitting down and eating meals like the rest of the world. But you may also be confronting the challenge of accepting a child's personal eating style. If you like to eat three square meals a day, and you expect your children to do the same, it makes sense that you may feel uncomfortable with a child who wants to graze, eating small snacks or meals all day long. Grazing behavior is, however, very common for kids of this age; they are small, have small appetites, and are not particularly interested in eating a lot at any one time. You can try to give her less frequent snacks to see if she eats more during a meal, but if her eating behavior does not change, do not despair. As her tummy grows, she will be able to take in more food at a time. See if you can get her to sit with the family for the meal even if she doesn't eat. Allow her to think of this as an activity by placing less emphasis on the food. In time, she will get more used to it. Also, as she matures, she will be able to sit still for longer periods of time.

4. The Sugar Baby

Q: My two-and-a-half-year-old has started to go to birthday parties. Until now, I have not allowed him to have sugar. Since having some cake at parties, however, he is refusing to eat some foods and keeps demanding, "Cookie, cookie!"

A: Make sure he fills up on healthier foods, but allow him to have some cookies. You can try giving him two or three cookies at a time and letting him put the rest in a special place where he can reach them. Give him a couple of options for when these will be offered again—tomorrow, an hour later, after dinner—this is your decision. Give him some choice about the time of day he may want to have the cookies, and set limits, as you usually would with temper tantrums or whining when he does not get what he wants.

5. The Picky Eater at Two and a Half

Q: *My two-and-a-half-year-old will only drink milk. Every once in a while he will eat chicken nuggets, but he eats no other foods. What should I do?*

A: At this age, many kids are enthralled by their expanding world and lose interest in eating. Rather than a conscious decision on his part, most likely your child's renewed interest in or reliance on milk is the result of his suddenly not having the time to eat. He's just off and running, very interested in his increased motor skills, and because of this, it's up to you to tune in to the best times to encourage him to eat. Make sure he is not too hungry and not too tired, or he will take the easy way out and reach for the cup of milk. Also, try to distract him by making eating a fun activity. Continue offering him a variety of foods. He will eat when he's hungry. You can also reduce the amount of milk you give him. Very often kids this age will rely on juice or milk to fill up because it's easier and they are interested in other things!

6. The Nonveggie Eater

Q: *My three-year-old won't eat anything green anymore, and I worry about her nutrition.*

A: If she is thriving and growing, she is fine and receiving her vitamins from other sources. If she resists vegetables, she may be more amenable to fruits, which are sweeter. You can also put veggies in smoothies, where she is less likely to see their offending color and texture. But don't fret too much; nutritionists I have consulted state that although vegetables are important, fruits contain many of the same vitamins. Many young children hate to eat vegetables. Continue to reinforce the idea that vegetables help her body to grow and stay healthy. And if she seems to be sensitive to their color or texture, take her grocery shopping. Let her look at the textures and colors of various fruits and veggies and choose those she likes. Don't force the veggies or she will be determined not to eat them in order to protect her right to make this decision. (You know how she is at insisting she wear that princess outfit to preschool!) You are still being a good parent even if you don't force the veggies!

7. The Beige Food Eater

Q: My two-and-a-half-year-old will only eat beige food. This is driving me crazy, and I really worry that he is not eating any vegetables at all.

A: This kind of food behavior is very typical of children around this age; children will often eat a nice range of foods, including vegetables, until the age of three, when suddenly they only want starch and carbs, such as french fries, mac and cheese, or other fairly bland foods that go down easily. This type of eating is very, very common, even if you think all the kids around you are eating their vegetables. Even if you and your partner are adventurous eaters, and you wish this for your child, he may not be that way, or at least not now. Don't get too worried about trying to predict the future.

If you are truly worried that he is getting no vegetables, cauliflower is beige and fits the color scheme. Try mashing it into pasta or mashed potatoes or mixing it with cheese. Let your child choose which beige vegetables he may like. Ask him about this preference, and take his response in a matter-of-fact way. Kids generally go through many food phases but always end up surviving their food preferences. If your child is on the growth curve and seems physically healthy to the pediatrician, don't worry and don't get too involved—that is key for picky eaters. As Dr. Michael Traister of New York City says, this kind of problem generally lasts no longer than a year. "The main health concern for Beige Food Eaters is a potential lack of iron, which can be addressed by offering Cream of Wheat cereal."

8. The Anxiety Snacker

Q: *My three-year-old is already eating emotionally. He is a pretty anxious kid; he had terrible separation anxiety at the start of preschool, and now I notice that whenever he is anxious he snacks nonstop. What on earth can I do?*

A: Although it is hard for parents to accept, small children do have complex emotional lives, and some are more emotional, sensitive, and, yes, anxious than others. Eating is, in fact, an anxiety buster, which is why so many of us use it to calm our nerves. However, you can help your child learn how to differentiate between eating to calm himself and eating for hunger. First, I would sit him down and say that you are going to be playing a game together. Explain that sometimes when he thinks he is hungry he really may be having other, difficult feelings. Reassure him that together you are going to figure out what he is needing more at the time. (Look at chapter six, Step Three, for ways to help him identify and verbalize what he is feeling.) Next, make sure he is truly not hungry, and again, look at Step Three to help him figure out the difference. Once he can identify what he is feeling, you will be able to find other ways for him to soothe, comfort, or distract himself. Perhaps he needs to be engaged in a favorite game, or maybe he just needs a hug. Try to help him understand that you know how he is feeling. If you treat him and his feelings in a matter-of-fact way, he will learn other ways to soothe himself besides turning to food. This will help him establish a healthy, long-term relationship with food and avoid any weight problems in the future.

9. The Picky Eater at Four Years Old

Q: My four-year-old daughter eats about six things—that's it. I know she is getting what she needs nutritionally. I also know I was just like her at her age. But I just can't handle the constant "You should get her to eat more!" from her grandparents and other parents. It makes me feel like they are questioning my parenting abilities.

A: It sounds as if you are facing what every parent faces: everyone else is an expert whose job it is to tell us what to do. But you are on the right track with your daughter. You know this is what you were like, you know it's very common for kids to inherit their parents' eating habits, and you know you need not worry about her. Trust your instincts and your understanding of your daughter; truthfully, you are doing more for her by respecting her eating habits (especially since they are not dangerous) and giving her room to figure this out herself without being overly involved. Continue to stay out of the way. You can continue to offer her other options, but if she refuses, let it go. You can also model your own enthusiasm about different foods, which often encourages kids to want to try new things. She may not begin to try new things now, but when her appetite kicks up and her body needs more food (often around age thirteen for very picky eaters), she will feel the freedom to experiment herself without the pressure of your agenda. Regarding the comments you get from others, the more confidence you have in yourself and your parenting, the easier it will be to let it roll off your back. Everyone is always going to have an opinion. It is yours that counts.

10. The Spurt Eater

Q: My daughter is four and a half and she's not a good eater. Sometimes she seems to live on air for two or three days! And to make matters worse, my husband and I differ on how to deal with her. I find that I am more patient with her than my husband is. I tend to let her eat when she seems hungry and leave her alone when she doesn't want to eat. But my husband thinks I am being too easy on her and that we are letting our daughter order us around.

A: First you need to determine whether your daughter is eating enough *for her.* Everyone eats according to his or her own body's needs: some people need to eat every few hours, while others can go for several days eating very little, then sit down and eat a lot. This is most likely how your daughter is. Use a food journal to write down what she really takes in for a week and notice if she has some days where she tends to eat a lot more than usual.

Next, keep in mind that she is eating to feed her body and not to please you or your husband. Make sure that you are communicating to her that she must know what her body needs and that she is the expert on knowing whether she is hungry or full. If she understands that it is up to her to check on what she's eating, she will feel and be more responsible in general.

If she is a light eater by nature and body type, and does eat when she is hungry, then trust that she knows what she needs. In fact, when she resists your attempts at feeding her, she is actually showing you that she is confident in her knowledge of herself. It's much more prudent to reinforce her positive self-regard than it is to communicate that she does not know what her body needs.

Frequently, young children who are very tiny and have their growth spurt later on are genetically wired this way. Were either you or your partner such eaters? If so, your daughter is simply following her genes. If not, perhaps there is someone else in the family your daughter takes after genetically.

In terms of working with your spouse, it's important to keep in mind that setting limits is an area in which many couples have different styles. One person is usually tougher than the other, and each person's style is usually related to his or her respective background and experience with food. Have a dialogue about your concerns and leave room for some differences. Talk to your husband about the pediatrician's opinion that your child is growing and thriving so that he does not have to worry about your daughter's safety, and explore his concern that she is ordering you around. Does he see this behavior happening in other areas? Is he worried in general about your setting limits? Is it that he ends up having to be the bad guy and saying no all the time, which feels unfair? You and your partner may have different parenting styles, which can actually be great for children to experience. If the two of you can arrive at a compromise, avoiding conflict every time an issue arises, your children will benefit from the give-and-take.

11. The Trouble Transitioner at Five and a Half Years

Q: *My five-and-a-half-year-old son has a terrible time turning off the television and coming to the dinner table. I have to give him many warnings, and it always turns into a screaming match during which I end up threatening to take away all his television privileges.*

A: This is a very typical reaction when children are glued to the TV set before dinner. It's as if they have been hypnotized, and even a child who has an easy time transitioning will not want to move! If your child tends to watch TV before mealtime, plan to turn it off a half hour beforehand and establish an activity to which he can then turn his attention. Suggest that he help you prepare the meal, set the table, or do another chore involved with the meal preparation. This will help him shift gears and dilute the hypnotic effect of the TV. You can establish it as a general rule; the structure will help give your child the transition time he needs and increase his ability to move toward mealtime.

12. The Junk Food Eater

Q: My six-year-old son asks to go to McDonald's every single day when I pick him up from school. I don't mind taking him once or even twice a week, but I worry about his eating that kind of food every day. He eats pretty well at home, but you hear such terrible things about kids and obesity and junk food!

A: Your son is at a stage when you need to pick your battles. He is not going to become obese from eating lunch at McDonald's every day, and if he is getting a good breakfast, or even just dinner, you don't need to worry about his nutritional intake. He is covered. Depending on how strongly you feel, you can experiment with taking him every day for one week. See what happens. Does he continue to ask for it the second week? (Or is it just the toy in the kid's meal?) Is he really eating all the food in the meal or skipping most of it and focusing more on the toy? (If so, you can figure out other ways to get him his toy!) If he is not a chronic overeater, having some french fries for lunch every day will not necessarily make him gain weight, but if you are uncomfortable with this plan, you can set the rule at once or twice a week and remain firm when he doesn't get what he wants. You can also explain your rationale to him, then find out what he loves so much there and let him know when and how he can get it. Suggest that he pick the day (or days) or time you go to McDonald's. You can give him some choice and still establish some limits. That is your right.

13. The Refuser

Q: My seven-year-old son refuses to eat with the family. He always puts up a fight and says he wants something different for dinner. What should I do?

A: There are several possible reasons for your son's refusal to come to the table. First, he may be having trouble transitioning from one activity to another. If you think this is the case, I would recommend that you institute a very structured half hour before mealtime, such as doing homework, preparing for the meal, or some other activity that shifts his attention to the kitchen and meal preparation. You can try what worked for another mother and her son. Her child had difficulty transitioning from the predinner activity he was involved with and would initially put up a struggle. But when his parents gave him tools to help him make the transition less stressful, such as signaling him that dinner would be ready in thirty minutes, then fifteen, and finally five, he gradually became more comfortable with the family rule of having dinner together. Eventually, he was able to sit with the rest of the family.

Second, if you think your son is protesting the food itself, help him pick one or two other options he can eat. Make them foods he can prepare himself or get from the fridge. For a younger child, three to six years old, you might have a shelf from which he can choose one or two foods so you don't drive yourself crazy.

If your child is telling you that he does not want to come to the table because he is "not hungry," you need to make sure he understands the rules or rituals that you have established around mealtime. If it is important to you that the family sit down and have a meal together, make that very clear by taking the emphasis away from eating. If your child insists that he is not hungry, explain that he is still expected to sit at the table with the rest of the family—even if he doesn't eat.

Next, reinforce to him that food will not be available all night long. If he is not hungry when dinner is served, he shouldn't eat. But he should know that the kitchen will be closed in another hour or two. (Again, make sure you are not held hostage and that your son does not manipulate or stall you at bedtime.)

If none of these options work, don't worry. If your child goes to bed hungry, he will remember that and might eat more the next day.

14. The Food Demander

Q: My six-year-old daughter is overweight (as per the doctor), and her nine-year-old brother is a string bean. They have always eaten differently. My son stops when he is full, but my daughter since birth has eaten and eaten and never seems to get full. Both of them are very active. What should I do? I don't want to say no to the food, and I don't want to create a complex for my daughter that will plague her with a life of dieting.

A: After looking at the nutritional content of your daughter's food intake over a period of two weeks, you need to ask the question, Does she really need more food or is she simply unable to detect her body's signal that she is full? There is nothing wrong with teaching children to stop and give their brains a chance to get the message from their bodies that they are full.

First, use the Hunger-Fullness scale (see page 124) to help her become more familiar with the idea and feelings of being hungry, sated, and too full. You want to remind her to teach her body to eat to the point where it is PER-FECTLY COMFORTABLE, rather than FULL. It is possible that she has become used to the feeling of FULL and interprets that as meaning she is done, which can lead to chronic overeating. She might just have to get accustomed to a different feeling in her stomach than she is used to.

Next, play the Waiting Game (see page 132) with her, so she can practice paying attention to her body's signals. After eating, suggest that she get involved in another activity to give her brain a chance to get the message of fullness from her stomach. Everyone's brain works differently, and the message the stomach sends to the brain, as well as the amount of time it takes to get there, varies from person to person. But your daughter may also need more time than your son to receive her body's signal.

If your daughter's overeating does not begin to subside, she may be eating emotionally, and food may be serving to soothe her. Your child may be having trouble separating true hunger from her other feelings. This could be a good time to help her differentiate her emotions from her hunger.

15. The Compliant Child

Q: My seven-year-old is a very easygoing child who has never given us any fight about food. In fact, we always thought we were pretty lucky, given that he has always just eaten what we have given him and never challenged us for not keeping sweets in the house. But now that he is in second grade, I have noticed that he has steadily put on weight. He has always been in the seventy-fifth percentile for height and weight, and now he is approaching the ninetieth percentile in weight. The only clue I have picked up is that he seems to be secretive about food and indirect when he responds to my questions about what he has eaten. What should I do?

A: Although his weight gain could be due to an impending growth spurt, my sense is that he may be hiding a change in eating behavior from you. Are you sure he has integrated what you've taught him about his body's nutritional needs? Or is he simply eating what you put in front of him to please you? Compliant children will often avoid asserting their will and instead hide their food choices from their parents. Your son might be eating the desserts or junk food from other kids' lunches. He may, in fact, be overeating these foods because you have not allowed him any access to them and he knows you disapprove. Talk openly about sugar with him and try to find out whether he likes eating sweet foods, even if he hasn't had them at home. Let him know that you will not be angry if he is eating sweet foods, and that you may want to figure out a way for him to have them in his lunch box and at home. You want him to be able to eat sweet foods responsibly; he can learn to do that under your roof, but you need to allow a certain amount of access. (For further directions on this please see page 106 in chapter four).

16. The Constant Eater

Q: My eight-year-old daughter is insatiable these days! She also has developed quite a pot belly, and she is always saying how starving she is! She eats very well nutritionally, she takes good responsibility for her body, and we have incorporated waiting, but there are still many days when she says she cannot fill up!

A: Many eight-year-old girls are entering puberty and put on weight in anticipation of starting their period. Additionally, they will put on some weight before their growth spurt. Nutritionists say that they get a lot of referrals of eight- to ten-year-old girls whose parents are concerned about their weight gain.

One of the things you want to look at is the kind or quality of food your daughter is eating. If she is eating well, eating when she is hungry and stopping when full, you want to continue letting her have access to foods—even if she is continually hungry. There are days and weeks when our children seem to eat everything in sight, and then they level off, or have a day or two when their appetites diminish.

You also have to remember that your child's body always seems to spread out before a growth spurt, and then lengthen out. (Suddenly the pants you bought just two months ago are above her ankles!) If your daughter is eating well and taking responsibility for her nutrition, keep reinforcing that she should certainly feed her body if she is truly hungry, and that her appetite is probably related to her body's needing to stock up on food for the onset of puberty and the growth spurt to come. As she becomes more comfortable tuning in to her signals of fullness and hunger, she will naturally become better able to take care of her own body. Be patient. Children's bodies go through a lot of changes. The important thing to teach your child is to manage food for the rest of her life so that her body can find its natural weight.

17. The Television Watcher

Q: My nine-year-old will only eat in front of the television. I am very uncomfortable about this, but I worry that if I don't give in she won't eat at all.

A: My intial response to this question is, "So what if she doesn't eat?" Your daughter is trying to manipulate you with her refusal to eat. She realizes that you care more about the way she eats than she does. It is your agenda, not hers.

First, you need to look at your family's eating style. How did your daughter begin to eat in front of the TV? Is she following anyone else's habit? Why does she need the distraction of the TV? Has eating become a stressful event for her? How often do you and your family sit down to eat together? Do the kids eat together on stools at a counter? Look at the family culture and your own values about time to connect. You can separate eating from television time. You are the parent and have the right to set up your family culture the way you want it. Don't let your concerns about food manipulate you! Let your child eat or not eat—as long as she comes to the table. That is connecting time.

You can also deal with this issue in another way: try establishing some occasions when it is okay to eat in front of the TV. Perhaps Sunday night, after the end of a busy weekend, or maybe even Saturday night, with a movie. You can also try using leverage by making eating in front of the TV a reward for doing her homework or carrying out other responsibilities. However you decide to establish parameters, you need to make sure that you are never held hostage to the threat of not eating. Children will always eat when they are hungry enough, so long as food is available.

18. The Dessert Sneaker

Q: I've been doing everything you say, and I let my nine-year-old son have a dessert of his choice every day. Yet, when my back is turned, he sneaks cookies from the kitchen. What should I do?

A: It sounds like your son is getting the idea that it would be problematic for you if he were to decide to have more than one dessert a day. Try to look at your own agenda and figure out why you are worried about his having more than one dessert. You need to give him more responsibility for making decisions about dessert, especially by his age. Nine-year-olds are very capable of figuring out how they are eating, and he needs to own more of the responsibility for his nutrition. It is not harmful for him to have more than one dessert a day; what is harmful is the growing tendency to eat compulsively that he exhibits by sneaking cookies. This behavior demonstrates that he is not responding well to the one-dessert-a-day rule, which suggests that you need to review your parameters and perhaps renegotiate the rule around desserts. If your son eats on the sly, he will take in more calories. Examine your own food legacy and concerns about giving up some control. As soon as you allow him more than one dessert a day, his compulsive behavior will stop. If you loosen up and give him more responsibility for deciding if he wants more cookies, he will probably end up eating fewer cookies.

19. The Dieter

Q: My nine-and-a-half-year-old daughter is fit and healthy and has always been an adventurous eater. But now that her friends are starting to talk about diet and weight issues, she has stopped eating. How can I convince her that eating less is not eating better?

A: Girls today are becoming very self-conscious about their bodies at younger and younger ages. Indeed, I have seen girls as young as seven or eight starting to diet, which can be not only physically damaging but also emotionally harmful. If your daughter does not have a weight problem and is becoming too concerned about her weight, it's important to address her assumptions about what happens when she stops eating. First, review the principles of healthy eating to reinforce her own confidence in knowing how much or how little food she needs. Next, go over chapter five, Step Two, with her so that she stays connected to her body's signals. Then begin to educate her about the fact that restricting food intake usually causes people to gain weight because the act of restriction slows down their metabolism. (This usually gets children's attention because it surprises them.) Also, help her to understand that being fit and healthy is based on the ability to eat all foods and never deprive yourself too much. Deprivation also leads to weight gain because it often triggers binge eating. Finally, talk to your daughter about her feelings about her body: Is she feeling less confident? Are there other things about herself she isn't happy with? If she focuses only on her body, see if she will talk more about these feelings. Does she feel that she needs to be perfect? Is it hard for her to make mistakes and move on? Talk about these issues. If she continues to not eat, definitely consult her pediatrician, a nutritionist, or an eating disorders specialist to avoid a serious health problem. A national organization called the National Association of Anorexia and Associated Disorders (ANAD) provides information and referrals throughout the United States, and, of course, you can also get a referral from your pediatrician. See Resources for further contact information.

20. When Dad Eats Junk Food

Q: *My husband can't stop eating potato chips, but he doesn't eat them in front of the kids, and he raises a fuss whenever they eat junk food! I think that sort of hypocrisy will cause our kids to really act out over food. What do you think?*

A: Your husband is probably afraid that since he can't control himself with potato chips, his kids won't be able to either. He needs to separate his own food attitudes (and behavior) from those of his children. If he fears that his kids will become "like him," unable to control their eating of junk food, encourage him to allow them to have access to junk food so that they can learn how to eat it moderately. Additionally, if he is worried about their nutrition, go through chapter four, Step One, so that you can help to alleviate his fears. Finally, it sounds as if he is also having difficulty letting go and trusting that his kids can learn to eat differently from him. The best thing he can do is learn how to eat the food he loves more moderately. If he reads this book, he may learn a thing or two about his own eating habits. If after doing the exercises in chapter one he is still having trouble separating his attitude toward food from the way he handles your kids, he may need further professional support.

Resources

National Association of Anorexia Nervosa and Associated Disorders (ANAD)

> national hotline: 847-831-3438
>
> e-mail: anad20@aol.com
>
> website: www.anad.org

> ANAD provides a national newsletter; referrals to therapists, health professionals, and inpatient/outpatient centers; support groups throughout the country and in eighteen foreign countries; presentations to schools and groups; and comprehensive information for teachers in middle and high schools.

National Dissemination Center for Children with Disabilities (birth to age twenty-two)

> phone: 1-800-695-0285
>
> website: www.nichcy.org

> The website provides referrals in your city and state for evaluation and services; primary purpose is for early intervention.

Center for the Study of Anorexia and Bulimia

> phone: 212-333-3444
>
> website: www.csabnyc.org

> Located in New York City, the Center is the oldest sliding scale clinic for the treatment of eating problems, providing referrals, outreach, and prevention.

Bibliography

Brazelton, T. Berry. *Touchpoints: Your Child's Emotional and Behavioral Development: Birth–3.* New York: Harper-Collins, 1992.

Bruch, H. "Family Background in Eating Disorders." In *The Child in His Family,* edited by E. J. Anthony and C. Koupernik, 66–97. New York: John Wiley & Sons, 1970.

Eisenberg, Arlene, Heidi Murkoff, and Sandee Hathaway. *What to Expect the Toddler Years.* New York: Workman Publishing, 1994.

Fairburn, Christopher, and Terence Wilson. *Binge Eating: Nature, Assessment, and Treatment.* New York: The Guilford Press, 1993.

Fichter, M. M., and K. M. Pirke. "Hypothalmic Pituitary Function in Starving Healthy Subjects." In *The Psychobiology of Anorexia Nervosa,* edited by K. M. Pirke and D. J. Ploog. Berlin: Springer, 1984.

Garner, David, and Paul Garfinkel. *Handbook of Psychotherapy for Anorexia Nervosa and Bulimia.* New York: The Guilford Press, 1985.

Hartman, Ann, and Joan Laird. *Family Centered Social Work Practice.* New York: The Free Press, 1983.

Haber, Ilg. *Your One, Two, Three, Four, Five, Six, Seven, Eight, and Nine Year Old.* New York: Dell, 1985.

Hendricks, Jennifer. *Slim to None: A Journey Through the Wasteland of Anorexia Treatment.* Chicago: Contemporary, 2003.

Bibliography

Herman, C. P., and D. Mack. "Restrained and Unrestrained Eating." *Journal of Personality* 43.

Hirschmann, Jane R., and Carol H. Munter. *Overcoming Overeating.* New York: Fawcett Columbine, 1988.

Johnson, Craig, and Mary Connors. *The Etiology and Treatment of Bulimia Nervosa: A Biopsychosocial Perspective.* New York: Basic Books, 1987.

Keys, A., J. Brozer, A. Henschel, O. Mickelson, and H. L. Taylor. *The Biology of Human Starvation,* vol. 1. Minneapolis, Minn.: University of Minnesota Press, 1950.

Kranowitz, C. *The Out of Sync Child.* New York: Berkeley/Skylight Press: 1998.

Leach, Penelope. *Your Baby and Child: From Birth to Age Five.* New York: Alfred A. Knopf, 1997.

Maslow, Abraham. *Motivation and Personality.* New York: Harper, 1954.

Minuchin, Salvador. *Families and Family Therapy.* Boston: Harvard University Press, 1974.

Moskowitz, M., C. Monk, C. Kaye, and S. Ellman, eds. *The Neurobiological and Developmental Basis for Psychotherapeutic Intervention.* New York: Jason Aronson, Inc., 1997.

"The Number of Overweight Youths Doubled in the Past Decade, New Study Says." *Nutrition Week* 25, no. 38 (6 October 1995): 1.

Samalin, Nancy. *Loving Each One Best: A Caring and Practical Approach to Raising Siblings.* New York: Bantam Books, 1997.

Samalin, Nancy, and Catherine Whilney. *Loving Your Child Is Not Enough: Positive Discipline That Works.* New York: Penguin Books, 1998.

Sandbek, Terence. *The Deadly Diet: Recovering from Anorexia and Bulimia.* Oakland, Calif.: New Harbinger Publications, 1993.

Bibliography

Spencer, J. A., and W. J. Fremouw. "Binge Eating as a Function of Restraint and Weight Classification." *Journal of Abnormal Psychology* 38: 262–67.

Tamborlane, William V., ed. *The Yale Guide to Children's Nutrition.* New Haven and London: Yale University Press, 1997.

Waterhouse, Debra. *Outsmarting the Female Fat Cell.* New York: Hyperion, 1993.

Wiedeman, G., and S. Matison, eds. *Personality Development and Deviation.* New York: International Universities Press, 1975.

Acknowledgments

There is no doubt that any project like this involves many people. While I can't thank everyone who has been part of this process, I am grateful and aware that without their giving me a moment here or there of questioning, or challenge, this book would not be what it is today. So thanks to all of you who have had any conversation at all with me regarding this project. All your feedback has been important.

Thank you to Brian de Fiore, my agent—you have said from the start, "Absolutely! Let's do this!" You have been part of the evolution of this book from day one in every way, not the least of which has been to connect me with my collaborator, Billie Fitzpatrick. Billie, your writing talent and organization of the material have built this book; but what has been most valuable to me has been your incredibly calm and soothing voice on the end of the telephone when I felt most frazzled and worried. You calmed me down at the most important moments and helped give me perspective, especially by helping me formulate my ideas and put what I do in my practice onto paper.

Tracy Behar, my editor, shared my vision and enthusiasm for this book. I appreciate not only your support but also the way you helped me rise to this challenge. Your calm voice and gentle but firm expectations helped me continue to think about this work and get the most from the material.

Thank you to all my readers, who took time from their busy schedules to read first, second, and third drafts; thank you for your support but most of all for your critical thinking and questions. Kathleen Giblin Ray—your spirit, straightforward and direct challenges to my thinking, and particularly your constant wry wit continually lift me; we've gone through it, girl! Jane Farr, M.D.—your take on these ideas has been wonderful; thanks so much for sharing your medical expertise. Thank you, Kelly Keane, for being a great reader from the mom and the English teacher perspectives!

Jane Guttenberg, M.D., and Michael Traister, M.D.— not only have you been extraordinary doctors for my children; you were also tremendously generous in putting time into my interviews and allowing me to "pick your brains" for your medical expertise and to understand what many parents struggle with in regard to their kids and food. Joy Bauer, R.D.—not only did you help me with the nutrition chapter and give me so much of your time, but you also gave me so much support and encouragement. I am so glad that we got to meet each other after all these years! You are truly a kindred spirit.

Jill Malden, R.D., C.S.W.—you gave me your time from the beginning. Your descriptions of your work and your stories helped bring levity to a serious subject—our children's nutrition and our own experiences with food. Thank you for all of the time you put into this project.

Helaine Ciporin, C.S.W.—thank you for helping me

begin to understand the issues around sensory integration. You shared your understanding of this subject so eloquently and were so willing to give me your time. Thank you also to Rachel Margolin and Terry Sash of the Life Start Program in New York City for helping me further my understanding of how to differentiate between kids with eating issues and kids who might have other developmental problems. You will have helped many parents to know when to worry, when not to, and when to seek early intervention.

Peggy Stern and Emma Ruskin—thank you for helping me develop my thinking; you also were part of this process, helping me to believe that, in fact, it does work! Thank you to all the parents and children in my practice, my seminars, and my workshops who allowed me to be part of their process and were willing to try out the ideas that form the steps in this book, and to show me the proof. You gave me confidence, and I am deeply grateful for your courage and willingness to share your experiences and vulnerability with me.

Karen Anderson—you have helped me every single day. Thank you for your friendship of so many years.

Ricky Barlow—you make my life work, helping take care of the kids, the house, and me. Thank you for your happy spirit, positive attitude, and ability to help me let off steam when I most need to.

Michael Fish—support doesn't even begin to describe what I know I get from you. You are always there for me and have been especially helpful during this process. The fact that you "knew" I could do this (as you put it; I thought at the time you might be slightly crazy) helped me through one of my most difficult, and self-doubting, moments. Dad, Aaron Fish—you always instilled in me the idea that whatever I put my mind to, I could do. Again, there have been moments when I questioned your belief in me, but I never stopped appreciating the guts you gave me to take on some pretty daunting things! Marlene Fish Adelson—you have been my advocate from the moment I was born. We have shared some unbelievable times growing up, and you have been the most amazing big sister anyone could ever want. Mom, Betty Molnar—you are my complete inspiration. I've watched the way you go through the ups and downs of your life, and you have instilled in me the ability to go through them as well. But equally as important, you have been my guide to being a mother; your commonsense, no-nonsense yet empathic approach is one I truly respect and believe in. I rely on you always.

To my children—without you this book could never exist. Nicole—you made me a mother. Your extraordinary tenacity, strong will, and determination have been evident from the moment you were conceived. You also taught me how to respect a child's sense of self and autonomy while providing the necessary parental support and direction. You have truly been my teacher. Sophie—your exuberance and gusto always give me joy; you bring those qualities to our family every day. And Lulu, you are a character! You continuously crack us up and have helped me to understand the truly picky eater. Each of you has been a victim of my theories and practices with food; thank you for letting me play with my ideas with you. And for responding so well!

And finally, to Michael Davis, my husband—first, I need to thank you for our children. Who could have imag-

Acknowledgments

ined?! Your extraordinary patience and tolerance have given us what we have. Support and understanding doesn't even come close to describing what you give me. And your continual dry and ironic take on things keeps me laughing and helps me take everything, especially myself, less seriously. There is absolutely no way I could have done this without you. Thanks.

Index

Age of child. *See* Developmental stage
Aggression, 77
Allergies, 78, 114
Anger, 6, 7, 142, 148, 149
Anxiety, 16, 141, 149, 174, 184
  snacker, 219–20

Babies, self-regulation in, 119, 121, 122
Babysitters, 26–28, 74
  dealing with, 205–9
  interviewing, 208–9
Backup foods, 49
Bad guy, 205
Balance, 117
Balance Sheet Exercise, 183–84
Bates-Ames, Louise, 51, 54
Bauer, Joy, 91, 94
Beans, 87, 91
Bedtime, 75, 205
  food issues at, 165–67, 195, 214, 226
Beige Food Eater, 59, 71–73, 77, 218–19
  tips for dealing with, 73
Belly-head connection, 119–40, 177
  communication breakdown, 121–24

Hunger-Fullness scale, 124–28
  satiety, 129–32
  taking care of their bodies, 134–36
  Waiting Game, 132–34
  "you are the expert," 136–38
Boredom, 16, 52, 55, 113, 142, 150–52
  hunger confused with, 150
  using food for, 142, 145
Bottle-feeding, 37, 38, 42, 44, 121
Brain, 41, 68
  communication between belly and, 119–40
Brazelton, T. Berry, 39, 40
Bread, 8, 10, 72, 91
  grain, 53
Breakfast, 7
  importance of, 94
Breast-feeding, 19, 37, 42, 92, 121, 156
Butter, 93

Calcium, 93, 98, 99, 101, 102, 169, 170, 179
Camps, diet, 6
Carbohydrates, 8, 24, 72, 87, 90, 91–92, 101, 102, 112, 117, 176, 178, 218

Carbohydrates (*continued*)
  complex, 91–92
  portion size, 91–92
Caregivers, 26–28
  dealing with, 205–9
  interviewing, 208–9
Cereal, 49, 71, 74, 91, 219
Cheese, 53, 72, 92
  sandwich, 53
Chewing, difficulty, 78
Chicken nuggets, 69, 72, 76, 92, 217
Cholesterol, 93
Ciporin, Helaine, 41
Clumsiness, 78
Cognitive development, 40, 41, 42,
  52
Comfort zone, finding your,
  191–213
Competitiveness, 149
Compliant child, 227–28
Confidence, 161, 162
  decision making, 162–64, 174
Constant eating, 229–30
Control issues, 5–7, 11, 19–20, 34,
  47–48, 68, 107, 124, 142–43,
  149, 193
  sugar and, 106–16
Cooking, 52, 197
Cravings, 176
Crawling, 42
Cream of Wheat, 219
Creativity, 151–52

Decision making, 137–38, 143,
  159, 160–88, 193, 231
  bad, 174–75
  Balance Sheet Exercise, 183–84
  confident, 162–64
  helping kids decide what they
    are hungry for, 175–80
  letting children make bad deci-
    sions, 174–75

Ouija Game Exercise, 176–78
  parameters, 164–73, 187
  parental role in creating confi-
    dent decision maker, 185,
    187–88
  practice, 180–86
  reinforcing nutrition lessons,
    179–80
Dehydration, 72
Dessert. *See* Sugar; Sweets
Developmental stage, 36–56, 80,
  192
  cluing in to developmentally ap-
    propriate behavior, 39–42
  eating style and, 60–61, 80
  eighteen months to three years,
    45–48, 60, 72, 74, 75–76,
    97–99, 195, 215, 217
  five to seven years, 51–54, 60,
    65–67, 72, 102–4, 134, 144,
    165, 168, 201, 223–28
  nine to eighteen months, 37–38,
    42–44, 95–97, 121, 195, 214,
    215
  seven to nine years, 54–56, 70,
    104–6, 130, 169, 180, 230–33
  talking to kids about food at,
    94–106
  three to five years, 48–50, 61, 75,
    99–102, 152, 199, 203, 219,
    220–23
Diabetes, 114
Dieting, 10, 11, 16
  endocrine changes in young
    women due to, 15
  girls and, 15, 55, 232–33
  See also Restricting food
Dinner, 7, 49, 108
  family, 210–13
  importance of, 94
Disequilibrium, 39–40
Distractibility, 58, 59, 77

Distraction, using food for,
142–43, 149
Drawing, 149
Drooling, 78
Dysentery, 8

Eating disorders, 70, 90, 201–2,
233, 235
Eating styles, 57–81, 192
Beige Food Eater, 59, 71–73, 77,
218–19
developmental stage and, 60–61,
80
Food Demander, 58, 60, 61–65,
172, 226–27
Grazer, 59, 75–77, 80, 196,
215–16
Picky Eater, 58–59, 69–71, 77,
78, 79, 137, 193, 217, 220–21
sensory integration problems
and, 77–79
Spurt Eater, 59, 60, 73–75,
221–23
Trouble Transitioner, 58, 65–69,
77, 223–24
Eggs, 91
Eighteen months to three years,
45–48, 60, 72, 74, 75–76,
97–99, 195, 215, 217
talking to kids about nutrition
at, 97–99
Emotions, 141–59, 162–63, 171,
176, 182, 184
boredom and, 150–52
development of, 40, 41, 42, 50,
52
don't try to fix, 143–46
eating for emotional reasons,
141–59
helping kids understand,
146–50
Hunger Exercise, 157

power struggles and emotional
distress, 152–56
red flags, 145
separating hunger and fullness
from, 141–59
Wave Exercise, 154–56
what hunger feels like, 156–57
See also specific emotions
Endocrine system, changes in
young women as a result of
dieting, 15
Energy, 81, 91, 92, 102
Enjoyment, eating for, 12, 129–30,
199
Equilibrium, 39–40
Erikson, Erik, 39
External vs. internal eating, 123

Family:
eating with, 75, 123, 194,
210–13, 224
refusal to eat with, 225–26
style, creating your own, 210–13
Fat, 87, 88, 90, 92–93
portion size, 92–93
Feelings. *See* Emotions
Fiber, 72
Fish, 74, 91, 176
Five to seven years, 51–54, 60,
65–67, 72, 102–4, 134, 144,
165, 168, 201, 223–28
talking to kids about nutrition
at, 102–4
Flexibility, 32, 104, 112, 117, 128,
186, 191, 195–200, 203,
210–11
importance of, 128
Food attitudes:
separating parental attitudes
from children's eating behaviors, 3–35, 200, 205
tape loops and, 12–21

Food Demander, 58, 60, 61–65, 172, 226–27
  tips for dealing with, 63–65
Food Pyramid, 87–89, 99, 113, 196
  chart, 88
Forcing food, 6, 44
Formula, 92, 121
Four steps of eating for life, 83–188
  belly-head connection, 119–40
  separating hunger and fullness from other feelings, 141–59
  talking to kids about nutrition, 85–118
  teaching your child to become a confident decision maker, 160–88
Fried foods, 10
Fruits, 8, 46–47, 72, 73, 88, 89, 91, 176
Frustration, 141, 148, 149
Fullness, 50, 52, 119, 120
  Hunger-Fullness scale, 124–28, 182, 227
  satiety, 129–32
  separating fullness from other feelings, 141
  signals of, 50, 67, 68, 122, 124–40, 142, 161, 181–82, 197, 226–27, 230

Gastric reflux, 78
Gender issues, 29
  obesity and, 29, 54, 55
Genetics, 33, 41
Gesell, Arnold, 39
Girls, 229
  diets and, 15, 55, 232–33
  endocrine changes in young dieting women, 15
  prepubescent weight gain, 54, 55, 229–30

Grains, 53, 87, 88, 89
Grandparents, intrusive, 205–7
Grazer, 48, 59, 75–77, 80, 196, 215–16
  tips for dealing with, 76, 80
Growth, 24, 29
  chart, 24, 71, 72, 81, 85, 94, 186, 192
  spurts, 30, 51, 81, 156, 222, 229
Guilt, 8, 31
Guttenberg, Jane, 72, 86, 124

Healy, Jane M., *Your Child's Growing Mind,* 160
Height, 24
Hormones, 15
  puberty and, 39
Hot dogs, 53
Humor, 5
Hunger, 52, 119, 120, 135
  going to bed hungry, 165–67, 195, 226
  Hunger Exercise, 157
  Hunger-Fullness scale, 124–28, 182, 227
  separating hunger from other feelings, 141–59
  signals of, 50, 67, 121–22, 124–40, 142, 161, 181–82, 230
  sleep interruption and, 124
  tiredness and, 158
  what hunger feels like, 156–57
Hunger Exercise, 157
Hunger-Fullness scale, 124–28, 182, 227

Ice cream, 114, 172–73
Imagination, 152
Impulsiveness, 78
Independence, 40, 46, 48, 49, 51, 53, 54, 55, 99, 168, 169
Individuation, 40, 46

Index

Intensity, 58, 61–65, 138, 143
  advice for handling, 64
Internal vs. external eating, 123
Intuition, parental, 79
Iron, 93

Jealousy, 149
Journal, food, 43, 74
Juice, 44, 109
Junk food, 7–8, 10, 12, 27, 30–32,
  52, 64, 107–8, 194, 199, 228
  eater, 224
  parental eating of, 233–34

Keys, Ansel, 14

Labels, clothing, 69
Legacies, food, 3–35, 200, 205
  family and, 9–12
Letting go, 198–200
Limits. *See* Parameters and rules
Loneliness, 16, 52, 141, 142
Losing interest in eating, 215
Love, and food, 11, 15–16, 27
Low blood sugar, 72
Lunch, 7, 210
  school, 53, 94, 135, 228

Malden, Jill, 94
Malnutrition, 86
Manners, table, 194, 212
McDonald's, 224
Mealtime, 76
  family gathering at, 75, 123, 194,
    210–13, 225
  See also Breakfast; Dinner;
    Lunch
Meat, 87, 88, 91, 93, 168, 176
Menstruation, 229
Metabolism, 13, 135, 232
  yo-yo dieting and, 14–15
Midnight waker, 214

Milk, 44, 91, 217
Moderation, 117, 129
  sweets and, 111–13
Motor skills, 40, 41, 42, 215
  development, 215, 217
  poor, 79

National Association of Anorexia
  and Associated Disorders
  (ANAD), 233, 235
Nine to eighteen months, 37–38,
  42–44, 95–97, 121, 195, 214,
  215
  self-regulation, 121–24
  talking to kids about nutrition
    at, 95–97
Nutrition, 85–118, 196, 215, 217
  developmental stages and,
    94–106
  at eighteen months to three
    years, 97–99
  at five to seven years, 102–4
  Food Pyramid, 87–89, 99, 113
  general guidelines for kids,
    87–90
  at nine to eighteen months,
    95–97
  portion sizes, 90–94
  reinforcing lessons, 179–80
  at seven to nine years, 104–6
  sugar issues, 106–16
  talking to kids about, 85–118
  at three to five years, 99–102

Obesity, 7, 26–29, 224
  rise in, 86
Oil, 93
Oreos, 114–16
Organic food, 8, 31, 195
Ouija Game Exercise, 176–78
Overfeeding, 26–28, 121–23
Overinvolved parents, 22–26, 137

Index

Over-justification hypothesis, 109
Overstimulation, 151

Parameters and rules, 162, 164–70,
    187
  being the bad guy, 170–73
  caregivers and grandparents,
    205–9
  establishing, 32, 49, 164–67,
    189–234
  finding your comfort zone,
    191–213
  keeping clear, 167–70
  partner differences and, 201–5
  questions to help you consider
    your, 194–97
  shelving rules on weekends, 198
  sweet, 111–13
  that work for you, 189–234
Parents, 1–81
  decision making, 163
  developmental stage of child
    and, 36–56
  family food legacies and, 9–12
  finding your comfort zone,
    191–213
  food legacies and, 3–35, 200, 205
  junk food eaters, 233–34
  keeping your child in perspec-
    tive, 192–94
  letting go, 198–200
  overinvolved, 22–26, 137
  parameters, 191–213
  partner differences, 62, 121–22,
    172, 201–5, 211–12
  role in creating confident deci-
    sion maker, 185, 187–88
  separating parental food atti-
    tudes from children's eating
    behaviors, 3–35, 200, 205
  tape loops, and effect on chil-
    dren, 12–21

underinvolved, 22, 26–29
unrealistic, 22, 30–33
Partner differences, 62, 121–22,
    172, 201–5, 211–12
Pasta, 8, 10, 72, 76
Peanut butter, 17, 23, 51, 53, 92
Pediatrician, 23, 24, 27, 30, 36, 38,
    81, 85, 93, 123, 219, 222–23,
    233
Peers, 51, 77
Perfection, 197
Perspective, keeping your child in,
    192–94
Picky Eater, 5–7, 10, 23–25, 58–59,
    69–71, 77, 78, 79, 137, 193,
    217, 220–21
  tips for dealing with, 71
Pizza, 53
Portion sizes, 90–94
Potato chips, 233
Potatoes, 8
Poultry, 87, 91, 92
Power, 48, 61, 99, 172
Power struggles, 5–7, 11, 48, 49,
    70, 71, 99, 100, 193, 230
  emotional distress and, 152–56
  partner differences and, 201–3
Prepubescent weight gain, in girls,
    54, 55, 229–30
Preschoolers. See Three to five
    years
Protein, 24, 72, 87, 90, 91, 98, 99,
    101, 102, 117, 168, 178
  portion size, 91, 92
Puberty, 39, 55, 229
Push-pull behavior, 51–52

Quick kid-friendly options, 53

Reading at the table, 194
Refusal to eat with family, 225–26
Regression, 40

Index

Resources, 235
Responsibility, 55, 62, 100–101,
    104, 110, 165, 168–70, 193,
    198, 229, 231
  parameters and, 164–73
  taking care of their babies, 134–36
Restaurants, 177
Restricting food, 7–8, 11–15, 176,
    232
  binge behavior and, 11, 12–14
  overeating induced by, 13, 14
  yo-yo dieting and, 14–15
Rewards, sweets as, 108, 109
Rules. *See* Parameters and rules

Sadness, 16, 141, 142, 145, 148,
    149, 174, 182
Satiety, 129–32. *See also* Fullness
Saturated fat, 93
School, 50, 51, 107, 135, 219
  lunch, 53, 94, 135, 228
  problems in, 79
Secretive eating, 31, 32, 33, 112,
    181, 228, 231–32
Self-regulation, 113, 115, 119–40,
    192, 226–27
  communication breakdown,
    121–24
  Hunger-Fullness scale, 124–28
  satiety, 129–32
  taking care of their bodies,
    134–36
  Waiting Game, 132–34
  "you are the expert," 136–38
Senses, 41–42
Sensitivity, 58, 59, 69–71
  sensory integration problems
    and, 77–79
Sensory integration, 41–42
  evaluating whether your child
    has problem with, 77–79
Separateness, 48, 51, 99, 203

Separation anxiety, 42, 219
Seven to nine years, 54–56, 70,
    104–6, 130, 169, 180, 230–33
  talking to kids about nutrition
    at, 104–6
Shopping, 197
Siblings, 47, 74, 81
Sight, 41, 77
Silly Supper, 32, 33
Sippy cups, 44
Sleep, 43
  eating habits and, 43, 121, 124
  going to bed hungry, 165–67,
    226
  midnight wakers, 214
Smell, 41
Smoothies, 73, 217
Snacks, 7–8, 30–32, 44, 45, 76, 80,
    123, 135, 194, 215
  rules, 45
Sneaky behavior, 31, 32, 33, 112,
    181, 228, 231–32
Soda, 10, 28, 64
Solid foods, 37, 42, 121, 123
Soothing, using food for, 142–43,
    144, 149, 184, 219–20
Sound, 41
  sensitivity to, 77
Soy, 73
Soy milk, 23
Speech, 41, 46
  delay, 79
Spock, Benjamin, *Dr. Spock's Baby
    and Child Care*, 85
Spurt Eater, 59, 60, 73–75, 221–23
  tips for dealing with, 74
Starvation, 86, 135
Stress, 15, 16, 94
Sugar, 7, 12, 17, 18, 28–29, 31–32, 47,
    48, 52, 61–63, 64, 101, 106–16,
    194, 196, 199, 201–3, 216
  issues, 106–16, 216

Sugar (*continued*)
  sneaking desserts, 231–32
  withdrawal, 28
  See also Sweets
Sweets, 8, 18, 28–29, 31, 48, 61–63,
    64, 88, 100, 106–16, 129,
    172–73, 176, 180, 194, 196,
    201–3, 216, 228
  dessert sneaker, 231–32
  last resort, 114–16
  setting parameters, 111–13
  as treat or taboo, 106–10
  when kids can't seem to stop,
    113–16

Table manners, 194, 212
Tantrums, 142, 156, 216
Tape loops, parental, 12–21
  effect on children, 17–21
Taste, 41
Teeth, 102
Television, 194, 223
  eating in front of, 194, 198,
    230–31
  turning off, 233–34
  watcher, 230–31
Temperament traits, 138
  eating styles and, 57–81
"Terrible twos," 46
Textures, food, 78
  extreme reactions to, 78
Therapy, 25, 200
Three to five years, 48–50, 61, 75,
    99–102, 152, 199, 203, 219,
    220–23
  talking to kids about nutrition
    at, 99–102
Tiredness, and hunger, 158
Toddlerhood. *See* Eighteen
    months to three years
Touch, 41
  sensitivity to, 69, 77

Traister, Michael, 46, 219
Trans-fatty acids, 93
Transitions, food, 65–69
Trouble Transitioner, 58, 65–69,
    77, 223–24
  tips for dealing with, 68–69

Underinvolved parents, 22,
    26–29
Unrealistic parents, 22, 30–33

Vegetables, 8, 46, 72, 87, 88, 89, 91,
    108, 109, 168, 176, 177, 208,
    218, 219
  children who won't eat, 217–18
Vegetarians, 89, 168–69
Vision, 41–42
Vitamins and minerals, 24, 47,
    93–94, 99, 101, 217
  multivitamin, 93–94

Waiting Game, 114, 132–34, 150,
    182, 227
Walking, 41, 42, 45
Water, 44, 47
Waterhouse, Debra, *Outsmarting
    the Female Fat Cell*, 15, 125
Wave Exercise, 154–56, 183
Weekends, shelving rules on, 198
Weight, 24
  gain, 30–31, 54, 65–66, 130, 134,
    137, 138, 180–83, 224, 226,
    228, 229, 232
Weight Watchers, 6
White food. *See* Beige Food
    Eater
Willfulness, 58, 61, 138

*Yale Guide to Children's Nutri-
    tion*, 90–91, 93, 119
Yogurt, 73, 92
Yo-yo dieting, 14–15